Autophagy

For Women and Men who Desire to Purify their Body, Lose Weight, and Slow Aging with a Natural Self-Cleaning Metabolic Process using Extended Water, Intermittent Fasting and a Ketogenic Diet.

Jennifer Cook

© **Copyright 2019 - All rights reserved.**

The content contained within this book may not be reproduced, duplicated or transmitted without direct written permission from the author or the publisher.

Under no circumstances will any blame or legal responsibility be held against the publisher, or author, for any damages, reparation, or monetary loss due to the information contained within this book. Either directly or indirectly.

Legal Notice:

This book is copyright protected. This book is only for personal use. You cannot amend, distribute, sell, use, quote or paraphrase any part, or the content within this book, without the consent of the author or publisher.

Disclaimer Notice:

Please note the information contained within this document is for educational and entertainment purposes only. All effort has been executed to present accurate, up to date, and reliable, complete information. No warranties of any kind are declared or implied. Readers acknowledge that the author is not engaging in the rendering of legal, financial, medical or professional advice. The content within this book has been derived from various sources. Please consult a licensed professional before attempting any techniques outlined in this book.

By reading this document, the reader agrees that under no circumstances is the author responsible for any losses, direct or indirect, which are incurred as a result of the use of information contained within this document, including, but not limited to, — errors, omissions, or inaccuracies.

Table of Contents

INTRODUCTION 6

CHAPTER 1: AUTOPHAGY PROCESS - CODE OF LONGEVITY . 9
- The Biology behind Autophagy's Anti-Aging Effects...................... 13
- Correcting Myths about Autophagy and Anti-Aging 16
- How Different Means of Turning On Autophagy Affect Anti-Aging 19
- The Newest Findings in Biology Concerning Autophagy and the Fight against Aging 23

CHAPTER 2: WHAT WE KNOW ABOUT AUTOPHAGY SO FAR 25
- Micro, Macro, and Chaperone-Mediated Autophagy...................... 28
- The Biology of Autophagy 38

CHAPTER 3: WHY INTERMITTENT FASTING 46
- Starting your First Intermittent Fast 57
- Protein Cycling during Intermittent Fasting 60

CHAPTER 4: KETO DIET 65
- The Mechanisms of Keto 71
- Keto: The Practical Walkthrough 76

CHAPTER 5: EXTENDED WATER FASTING 84
- Water Fasting: a Practical Walkthrough 91
- Inside the Mind of a Person doing a Water Fast 98

CHAPTER 6: METABOLIC AUTOPHAGY FOODS 102
- Eating Right for Autophagy 104

CHAPTER 7: METABOLIC AUTOPHAGY IN PRACTICE 122
- What to Avoid in Your First Fast 128

CHAPTER 8: AUTOPHAGY AND TRAINING TO BUILD MUSCLE 138
- The Health of the Individual who Exercises to Increase Autophagy 142
- A Note before the Conclusion.. 150

CONCLUSION 153

APPENDIX: SCIENTIFIC STUDIES ON AUTOPHAGY, INTERMITTENT FASTING AND RELATED SUBJECTS 158

Introduction

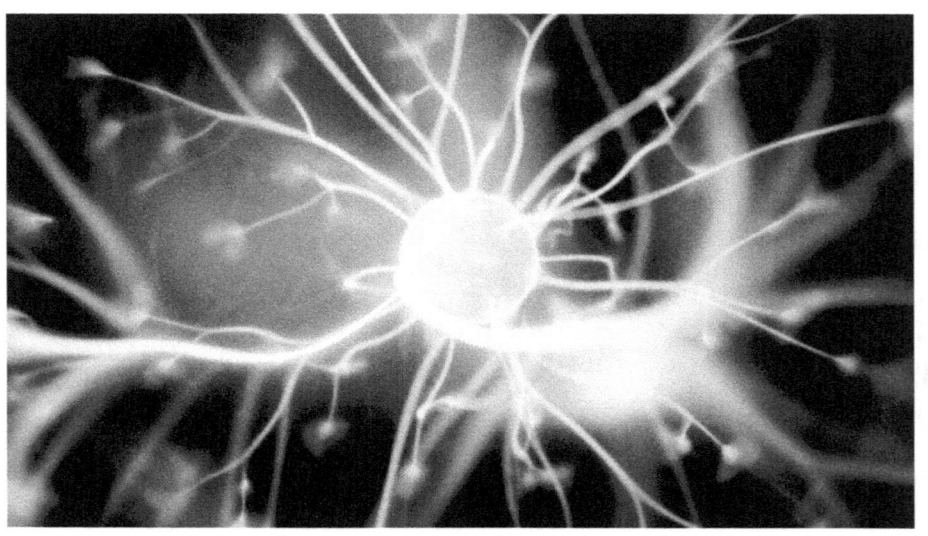

Congratulations on purchasing *Autophagy,* and thank you for doing so.

With the serious problem of obesity all over the world, not just in the United States, it is understandable that people are looking for a scientifically proven way to lose weight. Turning on autophagy in your body fits the bill perfectly. Read our comprehensive guidebook to the world of autophagy and how you can use its healing potential to lose weight, combat aging, and feel young.

Autophagy is at the center of the changes you can make in your daily life to see these effects. Put simply, autophagy is your cells' natural detoxifier. It is a natural biological process that has existed since the first single-celled organisms came to be on Earth.

Humans in the first world have lost touch with the process of autophagy because of the onset of industrialized agriculture and the resulting abundance of food. Not so long ago, we as a species went through long spans of time without eating. We didn't do this for the health benefits — we did it because we didn't have any food.

In the past, when people went through days without eating, our bodies started the process of autophagy in the cells. Since we did not have food in our cells for them to consume, our cells found alternate sources of energy to break down, such as damaged organelles, protein clumps, and various toxins. Autophagy gave us the twofold benefit of decluttering our cells and filling us with energy.

Of course, autophagy never totally went away. It is just that we don't go through it as much since we are constantly eating. Our book will teach you how to energize autophagy in your body so you can feel young, look young, and lose weight.

There are plenty of books on this subject on the market, thanks again for choosing this one! Every effort was made to ensure it is full of as much useful information as possible; please enjoy!

Chapter 1: Autophagy Process - Code of Longevity

As the years go by and you go through the natural process of aging, a lot of changes happen in your body. Your skin loses its stretchiness, you gain weight more easily, and you start to feel tired more often. Autophagy is your best friend in fighting against these processes so you can look and feel young for longer. Take the effect of autophagy on your skin. Turning autophagy on in your skin cells will allow them to produce more collagen, a protein produced by your fibroblasts, a type of cell in your skin.

Collagen is the protein that makes your skin stretchier and more youthful. It will put your cells in a routine of cleaning themselves out more so they can work more efficiently, making you feel more active and engaged with the world. This is just one of the benefits of higher autophagy in your body. The benefits of autophagy are innumerable, and it is never too late to learn more about them.

Until now, you've gone about dieting the wrong way. There are many diets that help you lose weight for a short time, but they're bad for your body, and they don't help you keep the weight off in the long term. This is what makes an autophagy-centered health routine so different from following fat diets. Autophagy is a method of keeping weight off your body while also considering your overall health — because you don't just want to lose weight. You want what is best for your general health.

There's also good news in the fact that for women especially, a lower BMI (proportion of fat to body mass) is a good indicator of your overall health. That might not be surprising to you; if you have ever been to the doctor after losing weight, it is unlikely they expressed concern over your weight. In today's society, in particular, many people struggle to keep their weight down. Doing so isn't just a matter of looking better — it is a legitimate indicator of your health.

Overweight and obese people have higher risks of heart disease, stroke, and more as they age. On the other hand, thinner people are not looking at these same risks.

Losing weight can only be good for your body, and autophagy is the healthiest and most effective way to do it. Autophagy will help you stay thin, feel good, and be healthy for years and years.

But so far, we have only talked about the health benefits that are immediately obvious. There is also a reduction of health risks that are not cosmetic, like youthful skin and weight loss. It has been proven that an increase in autophagy reduces your risk of Alzheimer's and Parkinson's disease. More autophagy also reduces inflammation, which will increase your overall health. There has even been research about the benefits of autophagy for cancer patients undergoing chemotherapy.

Studies have shown that cancer patients going through chemotherapy saw a reduction in the clumps of white blood cells that accumulate because of chemotherapy. Dead cells can be hazardous to your body if they are not cleaned out during autophagy. Since these patients fasted in order to turn on autophagy, their bodies were able to clean out the white blood cells and recover from chemotherapy sooner.

You can only imagine the kind of advantage you get if you are turning autophagy on as much as possible, and you aren't even looking at a major health risk yet. You may not have as big an accumulation of dead cells as someone going through chemotherapy, but if you have not fasted before and you don't exercise regularly, it is very likely that you have a lot of toxins in your body. This is because if you don't go through autophagy very often, materials like dead cells, dead organelles, and unused proteins start to pile up and make your cells less efficient.

Putting your body through autophagy doesn't just combat aging in ways that are immediately visible. It also greatly reduces your risk of long-term age-related disease. Whether you're looking to improve the quality of your life or the length of your life, making autophagy happen in your body will do it.

You can also feel relief in the fact that the book you are reading contains all you need to know about autophagy and how to best manipulate it for your health. After experiencing the life-changing effects of increased autophagy and consulting countless scientific journals on the subject, I know what information about autophagy you don't want to miss.

The Biology behind Autophagy's Anti-Aging Effects

Behind all the positive health consequences that come from autophagy is the biology that makes it work. As the pioneering biologist behind the biggest discoveries on the topic, Yoshinori Ohsumi underlined the importance of a process called cell recycling. Most books about autophagy tell us about the way our cells discard toxins, but they do not go into what our cells do with these broken down components.

It is not just toxin disposal that makes autophagy so good for us, but also cell recycling, so it's vital for you to know how it works. Scientists are still trying to understand some of the more intricate parts of autophagy, but they can tell us the basic mechanisms at play.

First, the cells must be put into a state of stress. This is where fasting and other methods of autophagy stimulation come in. These methods put your cells into a state of stress and activate autophagy. When they are under stress, autophagy begins with the structure called the autophagosome. The autophagosome travels inside the cell looking for things it can break down for nutrients, including all the things we have talked about so far: unused proteins, unused organelles, and other toxins that come from outside the cell.

The next step is where a cellular structure called the lysosome comes in. While you can think of the autophagosome as the transporter to the cell stomach, you can see the lysosome as the cell stomach itself. Back when the French scientist Christian De Duve discovered the lysosome in the 60s, we thought the lysosome was the cell's garbage receptacle; we did not know at the time that it was more like a recycling bin. The autophagosome takes all the materials it finds and binds with the lysosome, so these materials can be broken down for reuse.

There are multiple autophagosomes in your body, by the way, and the longer you are in a state of stress from starvation, the more you will have. More autophagosomes means more autophagy in your body. Research has concluded that you get the highest number of autophagosomes after 36 hours of fasting and that you do not see more autophagosomes after this point.

Of course, we are doing a little bit of simplification, but the next step is essentially the last step of autophagy. Even the microbiologists simplify things when they discuss autophagy because they don't know everything about this process either — the finer points of autophagy are still being worked out. The newest discoveries about autophagy are concerned with this third and final stage. In it, your cells take the broken down parts they obtained through autophagy and use them to build new organelles and protein structures.

Technically, this is not the final stage of autophagy, because by this time, autophagy has finished and your cells are no longer in a state of stress. This stage is the most exciting for people who care about advancements in science that have implications in health and anti-aging because with this stage we aren't just talking about detoxifying your body.

We are talking about using the fine materials gained from the detox for rebuilding cellular structures. When your cells use these broken down components to build new structures, your body has new, young structures at the lowest level, and this is a very exciting opportunity for your health.

When your cells have newly-built parts, they run more smoothly, live longer, and keep your body running efficiently. With autophagy, you get two great benefits in one: the removal of microscopic waste that would eventually turn toxic, and the repurposing of this microscopic junk into new, young cell parts that do a lot of good in changing your body into a healthy one.

To remember the stages of autophagy, think of the first stage as the autophagosome stage, the second as the lysosome stage, and the third as cell recycling. In few words, the process of autophagy involves the autophagosome collecting waste, the lysosome breaking down waste, and the cell using the parts left over to build new structures.

Correcting Myths about Autophagy and Anti-Aging

There are many misconceptions about how autophagy does its anti-aging work. Perhaps the most common is that its only health benefits come from taking care of toxins. Clearing toxins from your system is certainly a good thing, but autophagy goes far beyond ridding your body of harmful chemicals. Most of these toxins are not from outside your body, but they are materials like proteins and organelles that your cells used once and then no longer had a use for. These discarded materials start to take up space over time, creating clutter that slows down your cells. This is when they become toxins.

Some of these toxins cause even worse problems than congestion. The worst case is protein clusters that form in the brain. Neurodegenerative diseases like Alzheimer's become more of a concern as we age, and autophagy might be your best ally in fighting against your risk of these diseases. From a broader perspective, Alzheimer's manifests as "knots" and "tangles" in the brain that impair memory.

When doctors look at the knots and tangles with a microscope, they see that these irregularities are actually clusters of proteins that have built up over time. They are proteins that brain cells used at one point but later had no purpose. The protein clusters were not managed with autophagy, so they simply accumulated and started leading to serious memory problems.

Alzheimer's disease is the most extreme consequence that you can have from not going through enough autophagy. It is not the only consequence, however. Discarded materials like protein clusters start to build up throughout your body if you rarely go through autophagy.

In this regard, low autophagy leads to a low count of collagen, the protein that makes your skin youthful. Your skin cells can't produce collagen when they are crowded by cellular garbage. Similarly, you lose more muscle mass if you rarely go through autophagy because you are not turning on autophagy to repair the muscle tissue damage that results from physical activity.

From these examples alone, you can see that autophagy is more than a toxin-cleaning agent. Autophagy doesn't only destroy the bad (toxins); it builds the good (new organelles, proteins, and cells). Both sides of autophagy make it such a powerful anti-aging tool, one that was surprisingly given to us by nature.

So far, we have established that autophagy isn't just good for destroying pathogen invaders — it also destroys materials that become toxic when they linger in the cell for too long. In short, this biological process cleans out toxins from the outside and inside.

In the third stage, your cells use these broken down parts as ingredients to build new cells and cell structures. What's more: your cells have more room to build new cells and new cell parts because they freed up so much space during autophagy.

All these things come together when you find a way to turn on autophagy on a regular basis. Equipped with all this information, you know much more about autophagy than even your average fasting practitioner.

How Different Means of Turning On Autophagy Affect Anti-Aging

We will go deep into every method and how they start up the process of autophagy in different ways. To start out, let's just talk about what these methods are and how each of them combats aging in their own way.

The most well-known method is fasting. There are several different types of fasting, including intermittent fasting, water fasting, concurrent day fasting, and more. What makes fasting, so reliable is that you don't have to do something new, you just have to stop doing something that you are already doing. To turn on autophagy with exercise, you have to get into a new routine of working out regularly, and with the keto diet, you have to start a new way of eating.

In order to fast, you just have to refrain from eating when you would normally eat. We have already gone over the health benefits that come from autophagy, but with fasting, you also get health benefits from simply consuming fewer calories.

Back in the 90s, the idea of caloric restriction became very popular, and people saw improvements in their health from doing nothing more than eating less. There is even a great deal of evidence that mammals who restrict their calories live longer than mammals who do not.

This has not yet been proven to be true for humans, but still, restricting your caloric intake can only be a good thing. You get this additional benefit from turning on autophagy through fasting while also getting the benefit of autophagy itself along with it.

We have heard a lot of ideas about losing weight from nutritionists in the last few decades, but let's not kid ourselves: the main reason for weight gain across the planet comes down to people consuming a lot of calories without physically exerting themselves to burn them off. Fasting for any length of time will lead to consuming fewer calories, so you are on the right track for losing weight when you fast.

The next popular method of turning on autophagy is the keto diet. This method will turn on autophagy because it involves depriving your body of nutrients that it would normally consume for energy.

However, following the keto diet alone will not turn on autophagy because it is only activated when your cells are in a state of stress, and as long as you are sedentary or filling your body with any kind of food, your cells are not in this state.

That said, since the keto diet is so low in carbs, this style of eating will aid in turning on autophagy. I definitely recommend following the keto diet because the mistake many autophagy practitioners make is consuming a lot of carbs while they are not fasting.

Eating a lot of carbs will prevent your body from fasting for a long time because it takes a long time for your digestive system to process them. Not only that, but as you may be aware, it becomes harder to keep weight off the older you get, and you are significantly slowing down the process of burning fat when your digestive tract has a backlog of carbs. Fighting against this problem is the role of the keto diet in anti-aging and autophagy.

Next, there is the method of exercise. Studies have shown that resistance training, also known as strength training, is the most effective way of turning on autophagy, saying it is even more effective than fasting. The reason for this is that when you use your muscles, you are getting tiny tears in your muscle tissue that are repaired through autophagy.

The unfortunate thing is that exercising might be the last thing that people want to do, even though it is so good for their health. Like the other methods, exercise has its own health benefits that are separate from autophagy. Plenty of studies show that people who work out regularly have lower risks of all age-related illnesses, even those not related to the heart. If we are honest, exercising is probably the best way to fight aging.

If you want to get the most out of autophagy, you should employ all of these methods together. When combined, the keto diet, exercise, and fasting will give you the greatest benefits, both in terms of weight loss and in general health.

If you don't yet feel motivated to be as healthy as possible, try to think of the autophagy in your cells as an analogy for your personal health. If they did not recycle their cellular garbage, your cells would simply die after their organelles stopped working, or they were overcrowded with protein clusters and foreign invaders.

If you do not recycle your body's toxins by turning on autophagy regularly, your body will be over-encumbered with cellular garbage, and you will be less healthy as a result. If this analogy were expanded, you might even live a shorter life if you do not regularly clean out your cellular garbage via autophagy. Your cells try to live longer by using autophagy to combat their cellular aging — you should try to use autophagy to work against aging too.

The Newest Findings in Biology Concerning Autophagy and the Fight against Aging

Some of the recent findings about autophagy have turned out to be incredibly relevant to matters of personal health. It has only been in the past decade that we found out that Alzheimer's and Parkinson's disease are a result of a mutation in a gene that controls autophagy.

Let's step back for a second and define what we mean by mutation. As we age, the DNA in our cells becomes damaged from wear and tear. One of the genes in our DNA is the one that controls autophagy. When that gene takes damage, our autophagy is less effective because it is not getting proper instructions from the DNA.

As a result, when your brain cells create protein chains to do certain jobs, these protein chains become clusters that are toxic to your cells, all because these cells did not have undamaged genes from which to take their instructions.

Now you might worry that this gene damage as a result of age means that there is nothing you can do about it, but this could not be further from the truth. Your takeaway from this scientific discovery should be that you need to manually turn on autophagy as you get older because your cells' genes will not be as effective at doing it automatically. You can turn on autophagy through fasting, the keto diet, or exercise and get the same much-needed autophagy as you would if your genes instructed your cells to do it to themselves.

Chapter 2: What We Know about Autophagy So Far

Biologists used to think an organelle in cells called the lysosome was no more than a trash dispenser. It wasn't until the earth-shattering discoveries of scientist Yoshinori Ohsumi that we found out that the lysosome was the base of one of the body's most elaborate functions at the microscopic level. Put simply, autophagy is when your body's cells have no food from the outside, so they trap toxins, unused organelles, and discarded proteins in the lysosome.

The lysosome breaks down these materials into parts that the cell and build into something new. We have already covered these basic facts about autophagy, but it's good to review them to make sure we are on the same page.

When Ohsumi looked into autophagy with a tiny group of scientists, there were not many who were interested in the subject. Ever since winning the Nobel Prize, however, more biologists have woken up to how fascinating the subject is.

The group of researchers started out looking at autophagy in yeast cells in the 60s, and even today, they are still looking at yeast cells because there are still aspects of autophagy they do not understand. In science, it is best to use the same case to learn more about something, and for autophagy, they use the yeast cell as their case.

In an interview, Ohsumi has said he felt that they still only understand about 30% of the process of autophagy.

Even if they only come to understand autophagy 50% of the way, there is a good chance that these findings will be miraculous for people living with cancer or age-related diseases. The best part is that even armed with 30% of our modern understanding of autophagy, you can make changes to your daily routine that will help you live longer and lose weight. Still, it is exciting that scientists could find something revelatory by looking at yeast cells' autophagy that could change medicine completely.

We have discussed the fact that autophagy has been shown to be related to neurodegenerative diseases like

Alzheimer's and Parkinson's, but those are not the only diseases that it may play a key role in. There has been cutting edge research showing that when you put cancer cells (of a disease like neuroblastoma) in a petri dish with drugs that stimulate autophagy, those cancer cells are shown to have inhibited growth. In this case, the cancer cells were put together in a dish with a drug called apocynin, and the cancer cells had less growth because of the drug that stimulated autophagy.

This should be taken with a grain of salt because there has actually been research showing that autophagy can speed the growth of cancer cells as well — it just depends on the specific situation. But this is getting too far into the scientific details. The main takeaway for you is that autophagy plays an important, irreplaceable role throughout the body, and while your body is basically healthy, you cannot do wrong by stimulating it as much as you can.

In the following section, we will talk about the three kinds of autophagy that we know about so far. Before we do so, though, we want to clarify what we mean by "stress" in this book. There is a big difference between the kind of stress you put on your cell to turn on autophagy and the psychological stress that you might feel while you're approaching a deadline at work.

You do not have to feel psychological stress to turn on autophagy; you just need to put your cells under acute stress by depriving of nutrients or through exercise. If you do that, they will eat their cellular garbage in order to survive.

Micro, Macro, and Chaperone-Mediated Autophagy

Scientists know about three kinds of autophagy: microautophagy, macroautophagy, and chaperone-mediated autophagy. Microautophagy occurs in every cell of your body, so it is the most common. Meanwhile, macroautophagy happens only in specialized cells such as white blood cells.

Chaperone-mediated autophagy is the kind that scientists are studying the most because it has wide health implications that could potentially cure age-related disease or cancer. When scientists found out that Alzheimer's and Parkinson's were a result of failed autophagy because of damaged genes, these genes were actually instructions for chaperone-mediated autophagy. This specific finding brought autophagy to the attention of scientists at large. There are now many researchers looking into the intricacies of chaperone-mediated autophagy.

Microautophagy happens in every cell with a lysosome — that is, every cell in your body. I told you before that the autophagosome brings in cellular garbage to the lysosome, but that was just to keep things simple. The autophagosome is only used for macroautophagy. In most cells, only microautophagy is performed, and the lysosome simply pulls in the cellular garbage on its own, without the help of an autophagosome.

Microautophagy has several purposes. Every cell goes through this process to maintain equilibrium in the membrane, to survive when low on nutrients, and to maintain the size of organelles such as the mitochondria.

Scientists have looked inside the lysosome during microautophagy to see how exactly the materials are broken down, and they found that enzymes are sent into the lysosome to attack the toxins.

Once this process is complete, the broken down materials are used for fatty acids, amino acids, and so on. This is all part of the essential process all cells go through in order to survive, called the cell cycle. Becoming familiar with the cell cycle should help you visualize yourself as a cell that must constantly renew itself through autophagy, just as your cells do.

Now let's talk about macroautophagy, the kind of autophagy that is not seen in most cells, only in one with special jobs like white blood cells. This is the kind of autophagy that uses autophagosomes, which leave the cell to find materials like protein clumps, damaged organelles, and foreign toxins.

The jelly-like substance around the cell and inside cells is called cytoplasm, and the autophagosome has to take in materials from the cytoplasm and carry them over to the lysosome.

The lysosome is where the process of macroautophagy starts looking exactly like the process of microautophagy. When the autophagosome moves the materials into the lysosome, that part of the process is named by scientists' sequestration.

The other difference between macroautophagy and microautophagy is that in macroautophagy, the lysosome does not breakdown the materials. In macroautophagy, this is the autophagosome's job. The autophagosome binds with the lysosome to break down the materials.

The other name for macroautophagy is phagocytosis. The word phagocytosis is generally the term used for when cells run into a large particle from outside, and then surround it with the autophagosome to keep it under control. After that, the same procedure occurs, and the large particle is moved to the lysosome, where the materials are broken down.

The autophagosome is the special organelle that makes macroautophagy a little different from the other kinds of autophagy. Technically speaking, the autophagosome is not considered an organelle, but a vesicle. It is not truly an organelle because it is not a structure that supports the basic functions of a cell, but rather it is a tool that the cell builds to perform a task outside of the cell. As you know, the job of the autophagosome is to find materials to break down in the lysosome. It secures these materials with its double-membrane so they cannot escape.

The last major kind of autophagy is called chaperone-mediated autophagy. This is the newest type that anyone is aware of. In chaperone-mediated autophagy, the lysosome and the autophagosome do not work alone; they work with specialized protein chains. These protein chains have a job: to move particular particles into the cell stomach (lysosome). In other words, chaperone-mediated autophagy is not for getting rid of just any cellular garbage as in microautophagy. Chaperone-mediated autophagy is looking for specific particles using these specialized protein chains and bringing them into the lysosome for breakdown.

This is the kind of autophagy that scientists are trying to learn about the most since it is the most linked to certain diseases. It has been postulated that this kind of autophagy may be essential for the prevention of disease since it can use protein chains to find specific kinds of particles that can be broken down for specific raw materials, in order to build up specific structures. These specific cellular structures may be able to stave off disease.

So far in the lab, chaperone-mediated autophagy has been shown to play an essential role in repairing genes, in the breakdown of particles, and keeping the level of glucose at equilibrium. Chaperone-mediated autophagy is most similar to the process of microautophagy. The difference is that it does not break down just any content that it finds inside or outside the cell.

With microautophagy, the cell breaks down anything that is hindering its work as a cell. With chaperone-mediated autophagy, the cell is looking for specific content in the cytoplasm. The cell's genes contain instructions on what materials to break down in the process of chaperone-mediated autophagy.

With all this talk about how important chaperone-mediated autophagy is, you might be tempted to think microautophagy and macroautophagy are less important. But if you want to be healthy, lose weight, and feel better, it's important to turn on autophagy of all kinds because they all maintain the health of your body.

To be sure, chaperone-mediated autophagy is the most exciting kinds of autophagy to study for scientists. It is an established fact by this point that chaperone-mediated is highly linked to diseases that come with old age, especially as a result of neurodegeneration. There has also been a clear link made between cancer and a failure of chaperone-mediated autophagy.

As we have discussed before, this failure is the result of the degradation of genes that comes from aging. These are the genes that are meant to tell your cells to go through chaperone-mediated autophagy. When your cells do not have instructions from this gene to tell them to start chaperone-mediated autophagy, they do not, so protein chains build up and create toxins, particularly in your brain. This is why manually turning on autophagy through fasting, diet, and exercise is so important.

The proteins used in chaperone-mediated autophagy are called chaperone proteins, which is what chaperone-mediated autophagy gets its name from. Your cells use these chaperone proteins to bring waste materials into the lysosome that the genes tell your cells are important to break down.

We know the least about chaperone-mediated autophagy because it is the latest one that we have discovered, but it is also the most important to research for scientists because of its serious health implications.

Autophagy is constantly happening in your body, so when we talk about activating or turning on autophagy, we are not saying that it is not going on at all in the first place. When we say turn it on, we mean increase it. Your cells will go through autophagy no matter what, but the scale of autophagy is what is important.

The truth is that the cells in your body are going through autophagy right now, at this very moment, somewhere. But if you exercise, more follow the ketogenic diet, and fast, the amount of autophagy will go way up.

For example, someone who developed Alzheimer's is still going through autophagy, and they did before they started getting symptoms of the disease, but if they had stimulated autophagy before the onset of Alzheimer's, they may not have ended up getting it, because their cells would have been spurred to take care of the protein clumps that lead to the disease.

The research even shows that your cells reach a peak of chaperone-mediated autophagy after 10 hours of fasting. That means if you want to get some of the benefit of this special kind of autophagy, then you should aim to fast for at least ten hours, which is something that everyone is capable of.

That said, you still want to go further than that to unleash the full potential of this biological process, so you should ideally start with the ten-hour fast and work up to longer ones such as the water fast. We will get to the details of different kinds of fasts later on in the book.

It is quite exciting that chaperone-mediated autophagy only takes 10 hours of fasting to start up significantly, because it may be the most important kind of autophagy for you to turn on. Every type of autophagy will play an essential role in the cell cycle by getting rid of proteins that hinder the job of a cell. They will all involve reusing the raw materials from the dysfunctional proteins.

But chaperone-mediated autophagy is even more important because it purposefully and selectively gets rid of proteins that are harmful to your body, whereas the other types of autophagy will only remove these problematic proteins incidentally.

You can think of chaperone-mediated autophagy as the smart autophagy because microautophagy and macroautophagy do important work, but they only get rid of toxic protein build-up when they stumble upon it. In chaperone-mediated autophagy, your cells use the instructions in their genes to look out for and apprehend specific kinds of proteins that are bad for your cells.

Scientists have even named the special protein at the surface of the stomach that is used for chaperone-mediated autophagy, and it is called LAMP-2A. LAMP-2A is an abbreviation for lysosome-associated membrane protein. Part of the reason we know that this type of autophagy is so important is from research done on mice. One study found that when LAMP-2A was protected in mice, these mice lived healthier and longer lives than mice whose LAMP-2A was not protected.

If that doesn't convince you of the importance of LAMP-2A and chaperone-mediated autophagy, then I'm not sure what will. After all, it is just one protein at the end of the day, but it has such an outsized impact. The study suggests that we, as humans, should not underestimate the importance of autophagy in keeping us healthy. The importance of chaperone-mediated autophagy should not be underestimated either.

You may think there could not be possibly more good things about chaperone-mediated autophagy, but you would be wrong. There has been extensive research on it, and the findings are numerous. One of many similar studies showed that chaperone-mediated autophagy does not only have the function of breaking down specific proteins, but when done correctly, chaperone-mediated autophagy helps with glucose metabolism, and it can even help repair genes.

This is an especially important function since, as we have made clear, damaged genes can lead to a long list of diseases linked to aging. All of this is why scientists are interested in chaperone-mediated autophagy in particular.

In Parkinson's disease, in particular, researchers have found a connection with problems with chaperone-mediated autophagy. This problem happens because the proteins that are collected with chaperone-mediated autophagy bond with LAMP-2A too strongly, which causes clogging. It is clogging that leads to the protein build-up associated with Parkinson's disease.

You may be concerned that you already have a lot of protein buildup in your body, but no matter how far along this is, starting to turn on autophagy more will remedy the situation. Autophagy has numerous benefits: it will make your body's immune system better, it will prevent infection, cancer, and inflammation. These are just a few of the amazing benefits that autophagy has on your body as a whole.

The Biology of Autophagy

Your cells are the reason that your body is able to do anything. Even though they are so small that we can't even see them, you wouldn't be able to do any of the things that you do without your cells. Unfortunately, one of the most prominent features of aging is the degradation of your cells. Because of this, your cells' organelles are not as good when you are older.

The good thing is that you can turn on autophagy more so that aging does not affect your cells as much, and therefore they do not endure as much damage. When you do this, aging has less of an effect on you, and you will live longer than if you didn't activate it. If you are not turning on autophagy on a regular basis, your cells age and degrade much faster because you are not causing them to dispose of toxic elements as much, and as a result, they are full of toxins.

Your cells do not work nearly as well without autophagy: because of this, you are more susceptible to gain weight, having less youthful skin, having more inflamed pores, and having less energy. You are also more susceptible to diseases related to age.

As we have said before, the details are so complicated that even the smartest scientists are still trying to figure it out. But that doesn't mean it is impossible to understand it — in fact, everything that you need to know to be healthy using autophagy is actually pretty simple. Just like anything, there are specific methods to achieve autophagy at its full potential that will be explained throughout this book.

If you were just starting to explain autophagy to a friend, you might start out breaking down the word itself. You probably know that "auto" means "self," but you should also know that "phagy" means "eat." These are two roots from the Greek language, and together they create our English word. Autophagy occurs when our cells are put under a state of stress, and they eat parts of themselves that they no longer need or that even hinder the function of the cell.

The mitochondria is a prime example of this. The mitochondria is probably the most important organelle in your cell, and when your mitochondria aren't working the way it's supposed to, your cells will degrade their mitochondria and use them for raw material that your cells will use to build new mitochondria.

The mitochondria is not the only organelle that your cells do this for. All of your organelles are no longer useful after they degrade to a certain point, making it smarter for your cells to dispose of them and use the broken down parts to build new organelles. If they don't, organelles like damaged mitochondria would just be filling out more area in a cell than they deserve without actually serving a good purpose.

At times, you may think that I am overstating the importance of these microscopic processes in your body. However, these tiny events are far more important than you may realize. A mitochondria that is not well taken care of, whether from poor diet, lack of exercise, or lack of autophagy, can have deleterious effects on the body.

We have already talked at length about the relationship between low autophagy and neurodegenerative diseases, but it's important for you to know how big a part the mitochondria plays here.

A low-functioning mitochondria is closely linked to neurodegenerative diseases like Alzheimer's disease and Parkinson's disease. The best way to stave off a low-functioning mitochondria is by turning on autophagy.

It goes like this: you turn on autophagy through fasting, the keto diet, exercise, or a combination of these things; your cells build higher-functioning mitochondria to replace mitochondria that were taking a toll on the body; and finally, your healthier mitochondria runs the microscopic processes of your body smoothly and greatly reduces your risks of these neurodegenerative diseases. Of course, your mitochondria is not the only organelle that you have to think about, but it is the most important.

Sometimes the scientific terms can be overwhelming for anyone, so it is useful to think about autophagy in terms of an analogy. Whether you own a home or you rent a place, you probably have to deal with repairs someplace in your life. Even if you are on a lease for an apartment, you can deal with a broken vacuum cleaner or a broken dishwasher until someone from maintenance comes to fix it.

You don't have to know a lot about being handy to know one thing: it doesn't make sense to simply buy a new vacuum or dishwasher most of the time. Sometimes that may be the smartest course of action, but usually not. Usually, buying something new is too hasty. It saves you more money to try to fix the thing. You may have to end up buying something new, but it isn't smart at all to do that right away, knowing that you could potentially hold onto more money.

Your cells don't even have the choice to buy a new mitochondria, so they have to break down a bad one and use the parts to build a new one. They already have some supply of raw materials from broken down mitochondria if you turn on autophagy enough, so it is only logical for them to use them.

The cells throughout your body are quite resourceful. Autophagy occurs because they need to find a way to get food when they are not supplied with it. When this happens, they find nutrients in old things lying around that they don't need. That's where the discarded proteins, organelles, and toxins come in.

This process is the reason that humans can live for almost an entire month without eating. Your cells "eat" "themselves" (remember the origin of the word autophagy?), so for some period of time, they can go on without you eating food.

You may be surprised to hear that your system needs approximately 100 grams of protein on a daily basis. This is not an endorsement of a diet too high in protein, however, because you will be even more shocked by where the majority of the protein comes from: while approximately a fourth of it came out of eating throughout the day, the other three-fourths came out of autophagy.

That's right — most of the protein that cycles through your body doesn't even originate from the food you eat. It was already inside your body, and your cells naturally break it down for consumption. You might eat a slab of protein only once, but your cells eat that same protein multiple times over. It continuously cycles through your body in new forms.

It might start as a muscle cell; then, that cell's mitochondria is too dilapidated, so autophagy breaks it down and uses it as a new mitochondria. Later, that new mitochondria stops working efficiently, and autophagy turns it into a membrane.

The cells throughout your body can find protein nearly anywhere they go: in organelles, proteins that are no longer being used, and more. Without even your realizing it, your cells are building, destroying, and rebuilding these structures every day. Right now, somewhere in your body, one of your cells is constructing a new mitochondria with raw materials from a mitochondria it consumed during autophagy.

Any time your cells — or the cells of any plant or animal — go through a state of stress because of fasting or exercise, your cells start up autophagy. It is a cycle that is absolutely necessary for your survival as an organism. Without it, you could not keep on living.

I hope this chapter has provided you with a comprehensive but accessible resource to explain the biological mechanisms that make up autophagy. The rest of the book is dedicated to the lifestyle alterations you can make to turn your life around with autophagy. We will refer back to the science again from time to time, but only in reference to how to practically incorporate autophagy into your life.

Chapter 3: Why Intermittent Fasting

You have many things to choose from if you want to turn on autophagy throughout your body, but intermittent fasting is your best bet for several reasons. Methods like following the keto diet, exercising regularly and doing a full water fast work, but many people try these methods and give up on autophagy entirely because they can't commit to it in the long term.

IF (intermittent fasting) only requires you to restrict the eating you already do to a smaller window every day, and you still get to witness autophagy's anti-aging potential from this small change.

There is a serious risk of non-stop eating without taking a break by fasting. When you never fast, you are allowing the inevitable accumulation of toxins to damage your cells. This is why it is so important for you to turn on autophagy: so your cells can undo the damage that they endure from eating. Eating in itself takes a toll on your cells. The breakdown of food takes up energy. The particles that are not consumed simply take up space in your cells, making them less efficient.

Since it is hard for people to stick with regular water fasting without eventually dropping it completely, IF is the best way for most people to go. You can see the results that come from regular fasting, but you only have to make small changes, not big.

Do you remember what fundamental change in your body leads to autophagy? The answer is acute cellular stress. This stress can result from a variety of things, from starvation, exercise, and a sudden change from hot to cold or cold to hot. We haven't talked about the last one yet, but now is a good time to do so, because it provides a good illustration of why intermittent fasting is your best option.

You can actually turn on autophagy by simply stepping into a cold shower from room temperature — or vice versa, you could turn on autophagy by stepping into a very hot shower from room temperature, though I don't recommend it.

On a fundamental level, this works the same way as fasting and exercise because it puts your cells in a state of stress, just like when they are deprived of nutrients or when you give them microscopic tears to repair because of exercise. You could even step out of your house into the cold to turn on autophagy this way — or vice versa, step out of your room-temperature home into a scorching hot day.

Since this method of turning on autophagy fundamentally works the same as the ones we have discussed so far, why does it get so little attention? The reason is the same reason we are saving our discussion of water fasting for later.

Any method that achieves the result of autophagy is a valid method, but this book is not about turning on autophagy for a day. It is about turning it on basically every day so you can get the most benefit from it.

Some things seem interesting and exciting for a day or two, so much that you believe you will actually keep them up for longer. But then days pass, and you stop them completely. It is an issue of sustainability.

Ask yourself right now: are you truly going to step into a cold shower throughout the day to turn on autophagy?

You might consider it plausible right now, but if you did it for a couple of days, you would realize that you are not going to keep it up. At least, it isn't likely that you will.

Intermittent fasting (IF), on the other hand, is a different story. Just don't eat anything from Noon to 8, for example. This is an easy example compared to some intermittent fasts, but the point being made is that not eating between the same times every day is infinitely more sustainable than stepping into a cold shower every day.

Beyond that, it is doubtful that a cold shower will have the same level of effect as intermittent fasting. There has been little if any, research on the effect of sudden temperature changes on autophagy, but it intuitively seems to have less of an effect from a purely subjective standpoint. You will feel your body go into shock for a moment, but it quickly passes. We can fairly safely deduce that autophagy is not as stimulated from this momentary change as it would from the bigger change over time that intermittent fasting introduces. However, a splash of cold water before getting out of the shower is known to have its own benefits, such as making you feel more awake.

It is also worthwhile to note that the cold shower method doesn't come with the health advantages that come from caloric restriction, as IF does. Study after study demonstrates that IF helps people who follow it keep up energy throughout the day; IF helps people burn body fat; IF even lowers the risk of heart disease and diabetes. Some of these effects may be linked to autophagy, which a cold shower would give you some of the benefits of.

However, you are far more likely to keep up a routine of eating less every day than you are to keep up a routine of stepping into a cold shower every day. You will also probably not see the same level of health benefit if you are stepping into cold showers but continuing to eat unhealthy foods.

Now, let's dive deeper into the mindset one must adopt if they want to keep up IF to turn on autophagy.

You can't start turning on autophagy with a mindset of stress, because it is not necessary for you to be stressed. It is only necessary for your cells to be stressed. Think about it this way: while you are sleeping, you aren't eating.

Technically speaking, from the standpoint of your cells, you are fasting while asleep. Your cells aren't getting any nutrients at this time, after all. While you are unconscious, you don't feel any stress at all, but your cells do. This is why people have the highest levels of autophagy while they are asleep. They feel some level of stress because they have no food to consume for seven to eight hours.

All the studies are telling us that fasting is the best way that we can turn on autophagy. The experts in nutrition and health are also telling us that intermittent fasting is the best way to go about fasting since it is the most sustainable. Compared to our example of the cold shower, you can see why this is the case.

Even though this is true, your best option for getting the most out of autophagy is still using several methods of autophagy stimulation at the same time. You should make IF your main method of doing this, but you will only get more benefit if you use other techniques as well.

The reason intermittent fasting turns on autophagy is because your cells need a constant stream of energy. Being microscopic, your cells can't store vast amounts of energy, and they have to constantly create new energy.

The cell stomach (lysosome) degrades the toxins it pulls in (in microautophagy) or that the autophagosome brings it (in macroautophagy), and then the cellular garbage is changed into raw materials that are later used to construct new cell parts.

What we have not yet touched on is the fact that the process of autophagy itself requires energy. In order to understand how energy works in a cell for the process of autophagy, and to understand how intermittent fasting won't leave you feeling tired, you need to understand ATP.

Many people are concerned about starting to do intermittent fasting because they incorrectly assume that eating less will deprive them of energy. On the contrary, scientists are telling us that people who fast have more energy than people who are constantly eating.

People who fast a lot in order to get a lot of autophagy have the most energy of all. This is because, as we have said, your cells themselves are constantly looking for sources of energy. Unlike you, they are not able to simply stop. They have a never-ending job to do. This means that even when you are not eating, they have to find more materials to break down for energy.

People who fast with IF have higher energy levels than people who don't because their cells are "cleaner." You see, people who don't fast may be feeding their cells with new nutrients constantly, but the constant stream of new food leads to vast amounts of waste in the cells.

The cells are not equipped to break down this waste when they are faced with a constant barrage of food. They have no reason to clean out their dead organelles, misfolded proteins, and the like when they are constantly provided with new food.

This is why people who fast have more energy. They may not be giving their cells new foods to eat, but their cells still have plenty to eat from the past. They have previous proteins to consume while waiting for you to eat again. Your cells have no choice but to do this constantly in order to survive.

And if this seems odd to you, don't forget that your cells are already doing it without being triggered directly with fasting. While you are sleeping, your cells still need energy to keep going, so they are breaking down their unused proteins, organelles, and foreign toxins during this time. Turning on autophagy during the day is no different; it is simply better for your body because you are going beyond the bare minimum autophagy that you get during sleep.

Since IF allows you to go through a good amount of autophagy every day, you don't have to worry about not getting enough of it. The cells in your body get a healthy amount of autophagy while you sleep, and during your fasting period during the day, they go the extra mile to break down the cellular garbage in your body even more.

We talked about caloric restriction earlier in the book. Don't forget that you are also getting this benefit from intermittent fasting. You will be able to start intermittent fasting with a positive mindset because you can be certain that you are doing something that is good for you. You also don't have to go through the stress of trying something more extreme like water fasting, because IF is far easier to start and to continue doing.

So many people try a water fast (consuming nothing but water for 24 hours or longer) and feel completely burned out of autophagy stimulation afterward. If you don't want this to happen to you, your best bet is to keep autophagy on as much as you can reasonably do it with IF.

Ultimately, the decision of how to turn on autophagy falls back on you. I recommend you consider your own health factors when you make this decision. For instance, if you have issues with your lungs or heart, you really shouldn't be considering a water fast at all. As good as the experience can be for your body and mind, you still have to think about your own biomarkers. A water fast does take a toll on people with any organs that cannot risk further trauma.

That's why I emphatically tell you now: if you are thinking of doing a water fast and you have had a previous issue with your lungs or heart, just don't do it. It is not worth the risk to these major organs. Besides, you can get nearly the same effect from regular intermittent fasting. There is no need for you to do a fast as intense as a water fast.

You should not start a child or teenager on intermittent fasting, either. This is because individuals in this age range are still going through a period of growth. Theoretically speaking, anyone can get health benefits from turning on autophagy, but there is always a right and wrong context. This is an example of the wrong context for intermittent fasting.

You should also not do IF if you are a woman who is pregnant. Even if you have never had an issue with any of your major organs, your body is maintaining a delicate balance when you are carrying a child, and you can't disrupt that with IF.

Do not do IF if you have been diagnosed with diabetes. If you have diabetes, this should not come as a surprise. The amount of insulin in your body is too important to be tampered with through fasting, and IF isn't worth the risk in this case.

Finally, you should not start IF if you have ever been diagnosed with an eating disorder. Eating patterns are a difficult thing to change for anyone, but if you belong to this group, that may be especially true for you. There are cases of people with eating disorders who fell back into bad eating habits with the rationale that they are doing intermittent fasting. IF is meant to be a vehicle for good in your body, but if you use it as an excuse to fall out of doing good for your body, then it loses its entire purpose.

Truthfully, unless you have already gone to your general practitioner recently and they told you that you had no major health concerns, you should always talk to them before you make a major change in your eating patterns like starting IF. You want to be sure that your body can handle being deprived of nutrients for a set period every day.

IF may not be the most intense way to fast, but it is still a major change for your body, so you have to be careful with it. Only in the case that you are not a member of any of these groups should you proceed with IF.

Starting your First Intermittent Fast

We may have already gone into the mental aspect of the intermittent fast somewhat, but this is probably the most important aspect if you want to actually do it, so there is more for you to learn.

In specific, you need to learn this important lesson, a quote from Voltaire: "Perfect is the enemy of good." When this quote is applied to intermittent fasting and autophagy in general, it means that you can't be a perfectionist and do either of them well.

For example, if you want to do the intermittent fast and you completely forget about the fasting window and eat a snack, you might get frustrated and give up on IF completely. But in your first couple of weeks, you are bound to make lots of mistakes.

You are bound to eat during your fasting times. When this happens, you can't let it ruin the potential that autophagy could have in your life. It isn't the end of the world. You have to accept that you made a mistake and then keep going as if it didn't happen.

You are even bound to make mistakes after months of IF. No one is perfect. You may even do IF very well for months, get busy with a promotion in March, and fall out of intermittent fasting completely because of it. When that happens, you might feel tempted to give up on it too. You feel like you had a streak going, and you messed it up; it feels like you messed all of it up.

When it comes to intermittent fasting, you can't approach it with an all-or-nothing attitude. There will be weeks that everything goes exactly as you plan, and there will be weeks where it's as if you forgot everything you learned about autophagy. Remember: these blunders are inevitable. What will determine your success with IF and autophagy is your ability to get up and continue anyway.

There are lessons you can learn from your mistakes. If you keep eating during your fasting window in your initial week of IF, shorten your fasting window. You can always make it longer again later, but if you can't get yourself to fast for that long every day in the beginning, you can't let that stop you from fasting at all. Change your 12-hour intermittent fast to an 8-hour intermittent fast. Once you have a handle on the shorter fast, try to add a few more hours.

Perfect is the enemy of good. Perfectionism is the enemy of IF and autophagy.

We have a solid grasp of the mental aspect of IF now, so we can get more into the concrete details of what doing IF means.

You may be expecting there to be more to it than this, but besides everything else already included in this chapter, intermittent fasting involves exactly what the name suggests. You fast, but you don't fast continuously. You fast intermittently.

People who do IF first choose a number of hours that they want to fast every day. 8 hours is a decent place to start, but if this is too hard, you can go lower. Next, they pick a time during the day that this number of hours of fasting will go. For an 8-hour intermittent fast, you might choose not to eat between Noon and 8pm.

What happens next is easier said than done. You have to abstain from eating completely during this period of time in order to be faithful to your intermittent fast. If you can keep it up for a few weeks, you might want to extend the fast to 10, and eventually 12 hours. A 12-hour intermittent fast could mean eating breakfast at 8am, fasting until 9pm, and then eating dinner. Not everyone has to go this far, and not everyone has to go this far every day. What you decide to do is a matter of your own health situation and your own health goals.

Protein Cycling during Intermittent Fasting

It is time for you to learn about protein cycling. Protein cycling is a diet change that many people make when they do intermittent fasting. Basically, it means alternating between days of normal protein intake and low protein intake.

It is still important that you eat a normal amount of protein on the normal days because protein is an essential nutrient in your body. You need some level of normal protein every day, so your cells have it to build structures.

However, the low-protein days are important too. Having days where you consume little protein will further spur your cells to turn on autophagy during your fasting window. Your cells already have plenty of protein lying around as cellular garbage, so your cells can reliably use this as their source of protein on your low-protein days. (Don't forget the fact we learned earlier — your body processes 100 grams of it each day, and only a quarter of that comes from the food you eat!)

With all that in mind, you never want to consume lots of protein, no matter how important a nutrient it is. There is a very good reason for this. When you eat lots of protein, all you are doing is giving your cells lots of cellular garbage to clean out during autophagy. Your cells have to cycle between normal, non-stressed periods and autophagy periods, so it takes time for your cells to get rid of all of this excess.

When they take too long to do it, it eventually becomes toxic, as we have learned. Despite how essential a nutrient protein is, there is such thing as too much of a good thing, especially when it comes to protein.

When your diet is very high in protein, this hampers the progress of autophagy greatly. It does not hamper its progress as much as carbohydrates do, but it still slows things down. Instead of cleaning out your existing cellular garbage when you do IF, you will simply be cleaning out the junk left behind by all the protein you just ate.

Protein cycling gives us a great chance to discuss the importance of finding a balance between IF and a healthy diet. When you do protein cycling, you still need to eat the recommended amount of protein for a reason: it is an essential nutrient.

However, you can go too far in either direction. A lot of the foods people love contain protein, so it is common for people to eat far more protein than they should without even realizing it.

On the other hand, starving yourself of protein to the extreme is harmful, too. If you do this, you may experience loss in muscle tone that is usually associated with fasts more extreme than intermittent fasting.

To do protein cycling right, simply eat the recommended amount of protein every other day, and half or less that amount on your other days.

This is not only about protein, though. Even though IF is a fast meant for everyone, there are still ways we can take it too far. Take someone who makes their fasting window too long: let's say, 14 hours. That would mean they eat for an hour in the morning and then eat again for an hour before bed. This is absolutely unhealthy, and I recommend not doing this. It is still necessary for the body to receive some nutrients, even when fasting.

I especially advise against it because the IF is meant to be done every day. If you are fasting for 14 hours every day, that could have serious consequences on your body. With a water fast, you may fast for as much as 24 or 48 hours, but the difference is the frequency. Someone can do a water fast all day on Sunday and then go back to their normal eating patterns on Monday.

But if they do IF for 14 hours a day, there is never a time they return to their regular eating pattern. Their regular eating pattern involves consuming far too infrequently.

Maybe you are familiar with the concept of yin and yang from Taoism. The yang gives, and the yin takes. To find a balance between a healthy diet and IF, keep thinking of eating as yang and IF as yin. You need yang to fill yourself up with fresh nutrients.

When you are following IF, you do this outside of your fasting window. You need yin to cleanse your cells of the toxins produced from yang.

Too much of yang (eating) and too much of yin (fasting) both have negative consequences. The key is to find a balance between the two; this will allow you to get the benefits of both.

Put another way, don't let yourself believe that "extra" fasting will lead too better health outcomes. It won't. If you truly want to be healthy, you need to find the right about eating for your yang and the right amount of fasting for your yin.

Chapter 4: Keto Diet

Intermittent fasting alone will help you get rid of body fat, improve the quality of your epidermis (your skin), and change the way you think about eating. However, you can get the most out of IF by combining it with the keto diet. Keto and IF are a perfect match. The main characteristic of keto is drastically reducing your carb consumption, and this would also be a help to your body to start autophagy because carbs take a long time to break down.

If your main goal is to lose weight, keto and IF will also work together to help achieve this goal. Autophagy helps in this regard by cleaning toxins from your body, while the keto diet puts your body into ketosis, creating chemicals called ketones that aid in burning fat.

There is a good number of people who follow the keto diet but don't even know what autophagy is. This is a real shame because the two can work wonderfully together. While turning on autophagy is one of the best things you can do for your overall health, the truth is that a lot of people start following the keto diet for the sole purpose of losing weight. If your main goal with autophagy is to lose weight, then the ketogenic diet may be your new best friend.

You will have a lot of changes in your body if you follow a lifestyle of both turning on autophagy and following the keto diet, though, so keep that in mind. You can't expect to make such drastic changes without running into some things that you didn't expect. Both things have in common that people tend to feel slightly low on energy at first, but end up feeling more energetic once all the health benefits start to kick in.

All in all, autophagy is not something that can be reduced to a tool for losing weight, whereas the ketogenic diet can be, more or less. The entire purpose of keto is to deprive the body of carbs, causing it to release ketones that will then help you burn fat.

On the other hand, autophagy usually helps people lose weight because the means of turning on autophagy result in losing weight. Autophagy itself is about maintaining a well-balanced body, but fasting, dieting, and exercising are all the means of turning on autophagy, and all of those things also help you lose weight.

Changing your diet, in particular, will help you lose weight. When people learn how much exercise it takes to burn 100 calories, they tend to be very surprised. While exercise is an important part of the process for losing weight if you are already overweight, no matter your size, diet is always the most important. People who lose weight do it because they stop consuming more calories than they burn off with exercise.

The keto diet follows this rule, too. Being a change in the content of what you eat, it will ultimately be more effective than anything else. It also comes with the activation of ketosis, which is part of what makes it so popular.

Not only does keto involve eating foods that will keep you from putting on so much weight, but the lack of carbs will lead to a chemical process that helps you burn the fat you already have. Combined with autophagy-stimulating methods like exercise and intermittent fasting, you can't go wrong with using keto to lose weight.

Besides all the reasons I've already listed, I recommend doing intermittent fasting alongside the keto diet for one reason in particular. There are a lot of common mistakes people make when they decide to do intermittent fasting, and perhaps the most common one is not thinking about their diet when they are not fasting.

You could be entirely faithful to your 10-hour IF, but then choose to eat foods full of saturated fats and carbohydrates when you are not within your fasting window. I want to be very clear on this now: if you don't eat healthy when you aren't fasting, you really shouldn't be fasting in the first place, because you are wasting your time.

Diet truly is everything when it comes to health — or as the cliché goes, "You are what you eat."

If you are keeping up a sedentary lifestyle, eating foods loaded with sugar, salt, saturated fats, and carbs, and keeping habits like smoking or alcohol abuse, you might as well not fast in the first place, because it isn't doing what it should be doing for you.

At that point, you are using it as an excuse not to be healthy in other aspects of your life. If you keep up habits like these — habits that everyone knows are bad for your body — doing intermittent fasting isn't going to reverse all of those consequences for you.

This is where keto comes in. It gives you a template to follow for the food you eat when you aren't on the fast; that way, you are responsible for that aspect of your health as well. It will prevent you from running into this common mistake of thinking IF will cover for all your other poor health choices. And at the same time, you will get to enjoy all the other positive components we talked about.

In other words, following a keto diet while you do intermittent fasting is your best bet for keeping on track with your health overall instead of using it as an excuse to be unhealthy outside of your fast. You may not be ready to change your eating patterns to the keto diet at the beginning of your IF, but you can use this chapter as a guide for when you do.

Did you know that the median person living in the United States gets half of their calories from carbs? This country is also known as the one with the highest number of overweight and obese people — it can't be a coincidence that the health of their diet is one specific nutrient.

The keto diet combats this pattern of eating tons of carbs. If you follow keto, you don't eat more than 30 grams of it a day. As an added bonus, you keep your cholesterol low and eat unsaturated fats, both of which are good things for efficient autophagy.

Sometimes it's hard to remember something entirely without a vivid illustration from an example, so consider this: if you follow a diet low in carbs like the keto diet, your body will be finished digesting your food and start the process of autophagy in four hours. Alternatively, if you eat too many carbs, you slow down this process significantly. Your system will now take 8 hours to digest your food; 8 hours to begin autophagy.

Don't misunderstand: when you fast for 8 hours after eating, in reality, you are fasting for 4. And that's assuming you ate a meal low in carbs. Your body doesn't go through autophagy while you are digesting, and carbs take a long time to digest. If you didn't see how keto and IF were so complementary before, you must see it now.

In the next section, we'll go more in-depth on the mechanics of the ketogenic diet. After that, we'll give you plenty of advice on how to follow through with it.

The Mechanisms of Keto

Here, you will learn why keto is so helpful as an aide to making the rate of autophagy go up. At the end of the day, what you choose to eat and what you choose to do with your body are your choices alone, but I hope that we succeed in convincing you of coupling your IF with keto.

When the body breaks down glucose (the natural sugar from food), it uses carbs. The keto diet takes advantage of this and causes your system to produce ketones to replace carbs when you stop consuming as much carbs. Your body still needs to break down the glucose, so you are basically forcing it to do it by producing a lot more of a chemical that will help you burn body fat.

People who are on the keto diet are doing it as a means to the end of activating ketosis in their bodies. They do this by eating a far higher proportion of healthy fats than carbs. Since your body will always burn carbs before it burns anything else, depriving it of this chemical sends your body in ketosis, giving you a lot of ketones in your bloodstream.

You have probably thought for a long time that you need to watch out for fat above all else, but this is misinformation. It is not the amount of fat that you eat, but the kinds of fat that matters.

What happens for most people who find themselves putting on weight is that (1) they consume a lot of carbs, (2) their bodies burn through the carbs over a long period, and (3) their bodies leave behind tons of fat because they were so preoccupied with the carbs. Therefore, turning on ketosis has the twofold benefit of unleashing ketones to burn fat and to tell your system to focus on burning fat instead of spending all of its time on carbs.

Autophagy is more potent when you are on the keto diet because it is a diet consisting of few carbs and many healthy fats. Healthy fats are necessary for all parts of your body to perform their tasks, while carbs are substance that will slow down autophagy the most the more of it that you consume. Keto keeps you from eating foods that would seriously hinder the effectiveness of your autophagy, while also eating healthy, unsaturated fats that your cells can use to build new structures.

You can think of autophagy and keto as strongly linked using an analogy: intermittent fasting is to autophagy as the keto diet is to ketosis.

You use the first to turn on the second. You use fasting to turn on autophagy, while you use the keto diet to turn on ketosis. Ketosis is the central process and goal of the keto diet wherein your body produces the ketones that will greatly help to burn through your body fat.

We have already gone over the effects of autophagy and ketosis that you will feel, see in the mirror, and experience by living a life feeling healthier and living longer. However, you might be curious if there is a way you can measure your level of autophagy or ketosis in a more objective way.

While it does require some commitment, there is a way you can do this using the glucose-ketone index. Looking at this index will give you a pretty good indication of whether you are going through autophagy and ketosis (with this measurement, the two almost always go hand in hand). The first thing you have to do is purchase a blood sugar tester.

When you take a sample of your blood, be sure to do it when you are currently fasting. If you don't, you won't get a precise reading. This is because your body has a significant amount of glucose when you are not fasting, and the blood sugar levels that you read won't tell you anything about your autophagy.

First, you need to know the formula for the glucose-ketone index. When you draw blood for the blood sugar meter, you will see the glucose value and the ketone value. Before you do anything, divide glucose by 18; however, only do this if your blood sugar meter uses mmol/L. When the meter uses mg/dL, you don't divide by 18 or do anything. Then, you have to divide your glucose value by the ketone value. Finally, take this number and divide it by 3.4. Then you will have your glucose-ketone index.

You don't want your glucose-ketone index to be below 3. This is a level at which people have seizures or may be suffering from cancer. An index from 3 to 6 is usually a sign that you are obese or have diabetes. This is not a desirable glucose-ketone index either.

Finally, we have an index between 6 and 9. This is what you want as someone who is aiming for autophagy and ketosis. A person between 6 and 9 can easily lose weight or keep at the weight they are at. Finally, an index above 9 means you are not looking at a level of autophagy or ketosis that is sufficient.

Even though the index seems completely flawless and objective since it comes from numbers on a blood test, you need to take it with a grain of salt. A glucose-ketone index slightly below 6 doesn't definitely mean that you are obese, for instance. These numbers fluctuate somewhat, just like your weight. By the same token, having an index from 6 to 9 is not a sure way of saying you are the portrait of perfect health.

There are a lot of things that affect the level of your blood sugar, so an index like this is not completely dependable. You can't even know for sure if your index is where it is because of keto or intermittent fasting. Always use several indicators to decide if you are generally healthy. Ask yourself questions like: have I been losing or gaining weight? Does my skin look dry? How do I feel subjectively? That third question could seem to have less of an impact than the others, but you will be surprised how good you feel compared to before once you incorporate keto and IF into your daily routine. You have to pay attention to subjective experiences as well because your quality of life matters a great deal.

It should go without saying, but just to be clear, you always have to use more than one measure to assess your health. Continue to go to the doctor and be honest with them at all times. Listen to them and be open to what they say.

With all these caveats aside, the glucose-ketone index is a pretty solid way of figuring out if you are meeting your goals in ketosis and autophagy. You are probably in good shape as far as keto and autophagy if you are between 3 and 9.

Keto: The Practical Walkthrough

Before you get into this intermittent fasting and keto business, you are going to want to know what you should expect. Let's go over what happens over time for someone who does IF and follows the keto diet when not in the fasting window.

When twelve hours pass that you are on the keto diet, you already start the initial stages of ketosis. You are already burning through body fat without even working for it with exercise. As an extra perk, some of the fat that you burn through is converted into more ketones in the liver to burn fat.

By now, your body is relying on ketones for energy instead of glucose. This is yet another boon for autophagy since any significant level of glucose will stop significant autophagy in its tracks.

You will even feel a difference in how you think and feel. This is because your brain cells are using ketones for energy as well. There is a very good chance you will feel more clear-headed when your body is in this state of ketosis and autophagy. As a result, you may find yourself in a better mood.

Though the keto side of things is more about losing weight than overall health, you will be pleased to know that ketones don't create nearly as much inflammation as glucose does, either. For people who are trying to lose weight, inflammation tends to be high on the list of health concerns, so this is just another reason to do keto.

Let's fast-forward to 18 hours into IF and keto. You are now at a level of fat-burning and ketone-producing that you have not reached before. The amount of ketones in your body is much more than, probably, ever in your entire life.

When 24 hours pass on IF and keto, autophagy is seeing its best days. Since your system is running so smoothly because of the ketones, your cells are working tirelessly to dispose of waste materials, convert them into raw materials in autophagy, and then turn them into useful structures in the cell cycle.

48 hours into IF and keto, your ketosis is at its highest level. Autophagy peaks near 24 hours, while keto does around this point. Because of this, your growth hormones start reaching very high levels. Growth hormones have many benefits, including keeping fat tissue from building up and reducing muscle loss that comes with age.

Though we have already reached the acumen of performance from IF and keto, they still both do great work if you continue following them past the 48-hour mark. At 54 hours of keto and IF, your insulin is at its lowest level yet.

Keeping a low insulin is a great health goal to have because doing so hinders mTOR, a gene that stops autophagy from turning on when activated. As an added benefit, low insulin tends to go together with low inflammation.

Finally, after three days, or 72 hours of IF and keto, your cells are getting rid of poorly performing immune cells, and they make new immune cells to replace them.

Having young immune cells may indeed be one of the greatest non-cosmetic consequences of doing IF and the keto diet together.

So as not to mislead you, I will reiterate: the ketogenic diet is in no way required to turn on autophagy in your body. However, as you can see from this progression over 72 hours, the two lifestyle changes complement each other perfectly. It is almost like they were meant to be done together.

When you do IF with keto, the high level of unsaturated fats will cause you to go through even more autophagy than you would have otherwise. When you lose weight from these lifestyle changes, you won't have to deal nearly as much with the pesky issue of loose skin, because while keto burns your fat, autophagy will restore your skin cells after they move because of weight loss.

If you read all of this and still decide to do IF without following the keto diet, at least make sure you keep a low-carb diet. Remember: autophagy does not actually start significantly until you are done digesting your food, and when you eat more than a low amount of carbs, they take about 8 hours to digest. This is 4 more hours that your cells will not be going through autophagy.

While I have been going over all the good things about keto so far, there are certain warnings for you to keep in mind. For one, doctors warn that consuming a lot of fats — even healthy fats — can lead to damage to your gut. This is not to say to avoid fats altogether, because you need them. However, you can overdo anything, and healthy, unsaturated fats is one of them.

Originally, the ketogenic diet was conceived of as a treatment for people with epilepsy. Patients with epilepsy who tried this diet had half as many seizures as a result. Amazingly, they did not even see the seizures return when they stopped following keto.

The key to doing keto in a healthy way is the same as doing anything healthily: moderation. Despite what you may hear, it is not a good idea to follow a keto diet all of the time, no matter how badly you want to lose weight. Even epilepsy patients don't follow keto all of the time — what does that tell you?

Just stick with the original formula for keto: consume a lot of healthy fats, a not-low not-high level of protein, and a low level of carbs. Note that you shouldn't eat no carbs, because you do need them. You just don't need so much of them all the time. If you're feeling sick because of keto, that's a good sign that you should take a break from it, and wait to try again until you feel better.

Following the original formula for keto gives you sufficient protein for your cells to build new structures and sufficient calories to have enough energy. Traditionally, you follow a ratio of 4:1 of fat to protein and carbs. However, most experts agree that 3:1 is just fine. The best way to achieve this ratio is by avoiding starchy foods, breads, pastas, and grains, and sugars. You can still eat foods like nuts and some dairy products.

To follow the keto diet, the healthy way, listen to the following advice, and heed it. If you did keto for the past two weeks, you should be thinking about going back to a typical proportion of carbohydrates in your diet for a while.

It definitely isn't good for you to go without a normal amount of carbs for an extended period of time. It's just the same as I always say in this book: going too far stops being good, and starts being bad.

Just like people can take intermittent fasting too far sometimes, there are perhaps more people who take keto too far. Unfortunately, when we want to lose weight, we lose ourselves in that goal sometimes and start doing things that we know are bad for us. As an author concerned for your general health, you should know that I want you to think of your weight only as one part of the picture of your health. Losing weight is part of the picture of getting healthier, but not by any means. It is totally counterproductive to do unhealthy behaviors in order to lose weight.

To close, you want to make sure to stick the most important things about keto in your mind so you can make an intelligent decision about whether you will start following it. If you follow keto, you will start replacing the high volume of carbs that you eat with more healthy fats. You can think of "healthy" fats as synonymous with "unsaturated" fats.

Practically speaking, this means you have to stay away from the bottom of the food pyramid as much as possible: that's breads, grains, and pastas. It means avoiding beans, sugars, and snack foods, as these products are notoriously anti-keto.

By following this eating pattern, you will start ketosis in your body, since your system can't rely on glucose for energy anymore. It will start relying on ketones from your liver, a chemical that will greatly aid in burning fat.

Finally, the warning to remember with keto is not to let ketosis go on for too long. Two weeks is about the time that you need to start thinking about going back to non-keto foods for a while. But as long as you keep that in mind, you can harness the power of keto and intermittent fasting to lose weight and keep your body detoxified.

Chapter 5: Extended Water Fasting

Once you get into the habit of intermittent fasting, you might get more curious about more intense fasts like the water fast. You need to be mindful of what your body can handle with any kind of fast, but this is particularly true with extended water fasting because you will deprive your body of nutrients for as long as 48 hours at a time if you choose so. This chapter will tell you how to do your first water fast in a safe way, approaching it from both the physical and psychological perspective.

Your first-ever fast doesn't have to be a water fast, but I highly recommend that you try to do one at least once. You don't only do it for the physical benefits to your body; you also do it for the way it changes your mind.

When you go even 24 hours without eating in today's culture in which we never stop eating, it makes you see things differently. You start looking at food in a new way. You may even see things beyond food in a new way, too. Much like what happens when you do a keto diet for a long time, if you do a water fast, you are likely to experience a refreshing clear-headedness unlike you ever have before.

You might have run into the phrase "dry fasting" before, and while we're on the topic of these intense fasts, you should know this: it is completely fine for most people to go with only water and no food for 24 or even 48 hours.

But not only is going without water for this long bad for you (as in a "dry fast"), there is no reason for it. Drinking water does not stop autophagy the way that eating food does. If you did a dry fast, you would be dehydrating yourself for no reason at all.

A number of religious traditions include fasting for a reason. No religion is really centered on the health of the body; the reasons for fasting in these cases are usually for a renewal of spirit and mind. Whether you abide by the rest of the traditions of any particular religion, you can feel confident that there must be something to a pure water fast if people have been doing it for hundreds or thousands of years.

Like with intermittent fasting, there isn't much to say about water fasting as far as explaining what you have to do to water fast. If you consume nothing but water for 24 hours, you have done a water fast. However, there's still plenty more than that for you to keep in mind before you embark on such a feat.

First, you might wonder what the point of this intense of a fast is. Do you not get as much health benefit from a regular intermittent fasting routine? The simple answer is technically, no, you don't. While anyone can get more than what they need from IF, water fasting is for those who want to go that extra mile.

Consider this. If you are in the middle of your fasting window for your 8-hour intermittent fast and you eat a granola bar, you miss out on all of the benefits you would have gleaned from autophagy. That's because eating anything at all brings your blood sugar up, turning autophagy off. It may seem strange that even eating 70 calories would throw off autophagy so much, but it's how this biological process works.

Where does water fasting come in? You can get a decently potent autophagy process going if you are faithful to your intermittent fast, and you abstain from eating for a full eight hours. Earlier, we learned that assuming you follow a low-carb diet, you are still digesting your food for four hours after eating. That makes an eight-hour fast a "true" four-hour fast.

This is not to discredit the shorter fasts whatsoever. After all, your body's natural autophagy happens while you are sleeping, and assuming you don't eat four hours before bed, that's still "only" eight hours of autophagy. Combined with four extra hours of autophagy during the day, you are still going to extra mile to detox your cells and keep them healthy.

However, you might see the appeal of a water fast after seeing it this way. A water fast isn't something you do every day, of course, and not even every week, for most people who do them. Most people who do water fasting do it a handful of times every month so they can get as full an experience of autophagy for their bodies. Without water fasting, you can't truly achieve this level of autophagy. Most days, you have to eat, and after sleep, there are only so many hours in the day that you can turn on a high level of autophagy through fasting.

Occasional water fasts are an option for people who want to satisfy their desire to do a deep cleanse of their cellular waste. They continue to do intermittent fasting every day so they can get a regular cleanse, but every other week or so, they choose to do a water fast and truly get as much out of autophagy as can be gotten.

Don't make the mistake many people make with water fasting and drink coffee. For some reason, there seems to be this idea that you can drink coffee while water fasting. This is not true. Coffee breaks a fast. If you are doing a water fast, you can't drink juice, coffee, tea, or any drink with a substance that your body would have to process. The processing of that substance will cause autophagy to cease, completely ruining the whole point of water fasting.

There are writers on the subject of water fasting who concede that these drinks will stymie autophagy to some extent, but they say that at the end of the day, it doesn't make much of a difference. I beg to differ. We have a lot of scientific evidence of the effectiveness of pure water fasting — we don't have any evidence to back up a pure water fast, minus some coffee here and there.

Even a cup of coffee at the beginning of your fast can mess things up. Don't take the risk when you are already looking to get as much as possible out of autophagy.

Another common mistake is consuming flavored water during the water fast. Do not do this — again, the flavoring has something that your body has to break down. When your body breaks down chemicals, autophagy stops. You should even stay away from smells of flavor. It sounds bizarre, but even the smell of real or artificial food causes a parasympathetic reaction from your vagus nerve.

This reaction will actually keep autophagy from happening to a significant degree because it stimulates mTOR, a gene that will stop autophagy when activated. It may feel like there is such a delicate balance, but if you are water fasting to maximize the potential of autophagy, these are the things you have to consider.

Don't even take vitamins or supplements that purport to boost autophagy during your water fast. Not to beat a dead horse, but your body has to process that, and then autophagy won't start until it's done.

People who advocate for these supplements say that supplements don't have enough digestible chemicals to stop autophagy from happening, but they don't really know this is the case. They are just selling a supplement. (On a side note, there is no official supplement that is known to turn on or even aid autophagy at this moment, so you shouldn't bother shopping around for them.)

We went over what happens hour by hour when you combine IF with the keto diet. What happens over time when you start a water fast?

You will be happy to learn that in your neurons, the autophagosomes increase significantly after just 12 hours of fasting. Remember that this isn't really because of the "water fast," but because going much further than this length of time starts to be impossible for an IF practitioner, simply because of a lack of hours in the day.

The great thing about this is if you choose to make your IF fasting window include the evening right before you go to bed, and you rest well that night, you can still get to this 12-hour mark without even water fasting. Your brain should be feeling refreshed in the morning because of the deep autophagy activity its cells went through.

I hope I have sold you on water fasting, or at least got you interested on trying it later. Our next section will tackle the things you can expect during a water fast and how to prepare to do one.

Water Fasting: a Practical Walkthrough

Before we begin, keep in mind that the water fast is not meant for people inexperienced in fasts of any kind. If this book was the first thing to make you think about fasting, you should get used to regular intermittent fasting before you try this. A water fast under 48 hours is perfectly safe, but my reasoning is that you might get burnt out of autophagy completely if you fail to meet your own standards in the water fast, and we want to avoid that.

That said, it's ultimately your choice what you will do. Perhaps you read our introduction to the concept, and you are already all-in on this experience. In that case, make sure you read carefully and always think of safety and health first.

You should take a guess about what people usually notice first as a consequence of water fasting. It's an easy one, so don't overthink it.

If you guessed that they lost weight, you would be right. It shouldn't really be surprising that refraining from eating for an extended period of time causes people to lose weight. This shows that at the end of the day, losing weight is a matter of not eating so many calories without a plan to burn them off.

Your body relies on glucagon (glucose) after only a day of water fasting. You run through all the glucagon in your liver from just water fasting for 24 hours. When that happens, your system uses protein and fat for energy.

It is similar to how the keto diet causes you to start running on ketones, but instead of ketones, you burn through the protein and fat. This is yet another reason not to bring too much protein into your system — your system might choose to burn through protein instead of fat, which is definitely not a desired outcome.

Because of this, your weight drops very quickly. In only two days of water fasting, you lose up to two pounds every day.

This might make you feel tempted to water fast for long periods of time. There are certainly people who go longer than a day or two, and you can join them if you would like, given that you think you are ready. However, there has been some research about the impact of water fasting on autophagy, and scientists suggest that the number of autophagosomes in your cells caps around 36 hours of water fasting.

Now, if you water fast for longer than that, you are still going through autophagy for longer. Therefore, you are still getting this out of it. But in most cases and for most people, 36 to 48 hours will be your maximum for water fasting. Don't lose sight of the fact that you ultimately want to turn on autophagy for your general health. You are fasting for this purpose, not to just drop as many pounds as possible. The goal you set means everything for your health.

As someone who has done countless water fasts and remembers their early ones vividly, you need to keep in mind that the first day is the hardest. This is because it is very easy to spend the whole time thinking about food and what you want to eat. A sudden rush of cravings is very common for people on their first day.

When you last through the first day, however, you will stop having such strong cravings. They no longer have such a hold over you. Losing cravings is a really big part of water fasting because when you have them, they essentially give you the feeling of being hungry when you do not actually need food — you are just craving it. People are not good at telling the difference between the two. Once the cravings are gone, your health, in the long run, is positively affected, because you stop feeling "hungry" for these foods, you were merely craving all along.

Be cautious about the addiction to weight loss. Some people who get into water fasting, or even fasting in general, start having unhealthy habits once they realize how much weight they can lose.

But we have already gone over the dangers of pairing fasting with eating disorders. This time, I'm talking about the danger of inconsistency. Some people will do a water fast until they are happy with the number of pounds they lost, and then they go back to their normal life of consuming lots of carbs, not exercising, and so on.

You have to make fasting a normal part of your life if you want it to change your life. Too many people think they can exercise or fast a couple times a year and think it will make a difference.

Consistency is everything with autophagy. You can glean serious benefit from it if you water fast a few times a month, or intermittent fast every day consistently. You don't see any benefit from just doing it whenever you feel like it and completely forgetting about it the rest of the time.

We are almost done with the physical side of water fasting; then, we can get to the psychological side.

A large part of the purpose of the water fast is a detox. Since a water fast is so intense, you see intense health benefits from it. However, your senses are pretty attuned from the food deprivation while your body simultaneously goes through these shifts. One such shift is when you feel autophagy burning through your fat.

It is not a sharp pain like a knife, but it is far from comfortable, and you should be ready for it. Since it means fat is leaving your body, you are probably more than happy to feel this discomfort. Still, it's good to be aware of it, so you aren't surprised. You had tons of toxins inside your fats, and now they are all being released at the same time. You can't expect to leave them behind without this discomfort.

Losing the weight itself can also be uncomfortable. You may get a weird feeling in your skin. Be aware that these feelings are perfectly normal, but still be aware of the difference between this and being sick. If you do not go to dangerous extremes in your water fast, you shouldn't have to worry about this at all.

We have discussed the danger of water fasting when you have an eating disorder, but take what I am about to tell you with the knowledge that this is about something else. Sometimes, when people do a water fast for a while, they enjoy the high they get from it so much that they keep chasing after that high as if it is a drug.

Like I said, this is different from fasting for too long to lose weight. Here, I am talking about someone chasing a drug-like high that they get from fasting. This is something to watch out for, too. They keep fasting for longer and longer because the last fasting high didn't satisfy them.

Don't do water fasting if you are doing it for a high. Do it for the physical and psychological benefits. After reading the coming section about the psychology of the water fast, it will be easier to get your mind in the right place and make sure you are water fasting for the right reasons.

Finally, it's time for the technicalities of how you can get the water fast right. Although you can't consume anything with calories during this fast, everyone needs electrolytes in their body every day, and you might not have them in your water at home. For your health and safety, it's important that you still get electrolytes on your days doing a water fast.

There are a few ways to go about getting electrolytes. You can consume supplements with electrolytes with your water. However, the easier thing to do is just drinking water with a sprinkle of salt and a lemon to make sure it has electrolytes.

Next, there is the matter of what you put in your body when the water fast is over. There is definitely a right and a wrong way to break a water fast. The absolute wrong way to do it would be eating a plate full of bread when it is over. This would overwhelm your body with carbs to digest after making it accustomed to nothing at all for the length of the fast.

If you eat a lot of carbs to break a water fast, your blood will get a surge of insulin to break down the carbohydrates. Insulin requires a good amount of electrolytes, and while you should have electrolytes in your system, you definitely won't have a sufficient amount for the undertaking of digesting a bunch of carbs.

There is real physical danger to breaking a water fast this way. Doing so can lead to high blood pressure, a heart attack, and even sudden death. Thankfully, it is not hard to do things the right way.

If your first meal has to have carbs, make sure it's low carbs. But before you break the fast at all, make sure to get a thymine supplement into your system, as well as B vitamins.

The general rule of thumb for the meal that breaks your fast is 10 calories for every kilogram of your mass. You shouldn't eat a big meal, to begin with. Slowly introduce small, healthy snacks into your system. Also, be sure to have lots of water during this time, still using supplements or lemon and salt for electrolytes. It is good to introduce some healthy juice to your body at this time — all-natural, nothing with artificial preservatives.

Inside the Mind of a Person doing a Water Fast

The key to success and safety with the water fast is going into it with your goals clearly defined. Ask yourself right now, since you are pretty far into the book at this point: what are you doing this for? Do you want to lose weight? Do you want to look younger? Do you want to live longer?

While it's true that autophagy achieves all three for you, you still need to have a purpose for autophagy that is for you and you alone. If you don't, you won't be very likely to change entire aspects of your lifestyle for it. Once you have a well-defined purpose for something, all the rest starts to fall into place, because you know what you want to do.

The opposite of that is when you don't have a well-defined purpose at all, and you give up easily. If you don't know why you're doing something, it is very easy for you to give up on it. You don't even have a point in continuing with it, so why wouldn't you?

It is very easy to start things. Anyone can start a 300-word novel. Anyone can start a sculpture. What makes you accomplished is when you can start something and finish it. Autophagy and water fasting is no different. If you have a clear reason you want to see through your first water fast to the end, you will be far less likely to fall out of it.

Having your goal in mind isn't just a preventive measure against giving up; it's almost a way for you to do things the right way. If you are in the middle of a water fast, you might be tempted to get a snack, even though you know it ruins the purpose of the entire fast. When you already know your goal for water fasting, though, you are a lot less likely to fall for temptations like these.

You can tell yourself, "I am fasting to lose weight. I won't lose weight if I add more food into my stomach during this fast, so I'm not going to cheat on the fast with that cookie."

Alternatively, if you went into your water fast without a goal like this, things would probably go a lot different. You would see the cookie and say, "Well, it is my first-day fasting. I can do things the correct way next time." Since you don't have a clear reason for water fasting, there just isn't that emotional weight to cheating on the fast that there otherwise would be.

A second crucial but often overlooked part of the mindset of someone who succeeds in the water fast is knowledge of fasts and autophagy. Plenty of people believe they know things about these topics, so much that they actually do fasting the way they believe is correct, whether it is right or not.

Fortunately, you have this whole book of easy-to-understand information about fasting and autophagy. You could return to it if you need to know more, but chances are, you are absorbing it so well that it isn't even necessary. You already have this second crucial part of the mindset covered.

Finally, there is the third and last part of the mindset required to succeed in a water fast, and it is adaptability. You have lots of goals that propelled you to do a water fast in the first place, but the one that will carry the fate of all the others is your adaptability to a new, healthier way of living. This mental aspect will determine if you continue water fasting a few times a month, or if it is just something you do one time and never again.

You will get some health benefits from the autophagy that comes from water fasting one time, but these benefits are pointless if you don't keep it up. That's why it's so crucial that you adapt well to the new habits you formed and do it again in a few weeks.

Chapter 6: Metabolic Autophagy Foods

You can find many writers who will sell you supplements claiming to boost autophagy. While the ingredients in these supplements may be what you are looking for, there is one crucial thing to know: getting these nutrients from supplements will not have the same benefit as from consuming them in your food.

The famous omega-3 fats from fish are a prime example. There is an overwhelming amount of evidence to suggest the great benefit of getting these healthy fats from fish, but none to suggest you will get the same reward by getting them from a supplement. To save your wallet and your health, this chapter will walk you through many tips like this so you can eat the right foods while using techniques to turn on autophagy.

There are always people out there trying to tell you there is an easy way of doing things. I am not here to tell you that turning on autophagy has to be hard, because it doesn't. But any time someone tells you that you can make autophagy happen by taking a supplement that they are selling you, you can know that their agenda is to sell their product, not to tell you the truth about autophagy.

That said, pharmacists are working on such a product. We are not there yet, though, and anyone claiming that we are is lying.

People are always going to be resistant to doing things the slow way. We are always looking for shortcuts so we don't have to put in the time or effort. There rarely is a true, easy way — however, that doesn't mean it has to be complicated. Turning on autophagy is simple, but not easy.

After all, you only have to eat the right foods, fast at some level, get plenty of sleep, and exercise. It's not as if these concepts are hard to understand; it is just that action is always harder than talk. Any time someone tells you that you can turn on autophagy without doing these things is not telling the truth. This could be true in the future, but we are not there yet.

These truths may be a bit hard to swallow at first, but as you get into the right habits that turn on autophagy, you will realize that it is completely true when I say this stuff is simple, but not easy.

With all that in mind, you are ready to learn about what you should eat to get the most out of your autophagy.

Eating Right for Autophagy

It is totally understandable to be overwhelmed by this information at first, so don't be shy about reading through it for mere familiarity at first. This is information that you would be best off referring back to when you need it.

The most basic principle of eating right for autophagy is making sure you are getting significant autophagy in every organ in your body. So far, we have only talked about autophagy in terms of cells, but that is not what our goal is at the end of the day. We want the autophagy to aim for the betterment of our heart, liver, and lungs most of all. There are foods that will help autophagy target these organs, and we are about to go over them.

While there are no supplements that turn on autophagy directly, there are supplements that help you target the betterment of these vital organs. However, they are only effective if they are combined with a full of nutrients and vitamins. In other words, there is no point in taking a bunch of supplements if you are not eating healthy as well. It is no different from when we said you can't expect to fast to turn on autophagy and have it counteract all the other unhealthy habits you might have like drinking heavily, smoking, overeating, and so forth. The principle of consistency in autophagy requires that you keep a regular schedule of autophagy stimulating habits while also being healthy in other aspects at the same time.

You learned a bit about healthy fats in our chapter about the ketogenic diet, but there is still more for you to learn. Omega-3 fats are an important fat for you to get, but like we said, there is no evidence that you will get the same benefit from it if you are only taking supplements that give you Omega-3 fats — and on the other side of things, there is plenty of evidence that getting Omega-3 fats from actual food has lots of benefits.

This idea applies to supplements in general. When it comes down to it, taking lots of supplements may be marginally better than not taking any at all. But if at all possible, you should get these nutrients and vitamins from actual food and not from a supplement.

You may think that you can find Omega-3 fats in the meat aisle at your local grocery store, which sadly may not be the case. This is because a lot of the meat at grocery stores tends to be sourced from factory farms. Animals that are raised in these farms are not grass-fed in a normal environment, and they are altered with artificial chemicals. Since they are not feeding on natural food like grass, you are not getting these nutrients indirectly as you should. Instead, you are getting artificial chemicals that these animals are fed to make them bigger and thus more profitable for the farm.

They may be expensive, but health grocery stores should be an option that you strongly consider if you want to take autophagy and your body's health seriously. These are places where you can buy meat that does not come from factory farms, and that will have the Omega-3 fats that they should because of it.

Next, we get to the matter of vegetables. Vegetables seem to be the exercise of the food pyramid: everyone knows that it is good, but many people don't like to eat it. If this describes you, you might want to think about using a blender and blending vegetables with fruit so you will eat them.

There are vitamins and nutrients in vegetables that you won't get anywhere else, so it is worthwhile to get yourself to eat them any way that you can. However, be warned that you shouldn't add a lot of fruit, because fruit is high in sugar, which raises your glucose, which prevents autophagy from happening to a significant degree.

You should also think about drinking more green tea. Green tea does a lot of good in making your AMPK go up. While mTOR is the gene that stops autophagy in its tracks, AMPK is the opposite: when stimulated, AMPK will tell your autophagy to turn on.

Green tea makes AMPK go up (and therefore helps to turn on autophagy) particularly well when you couple it with turmeric. Turmeric is actually even more effective in stimulating AMPK, but when you use it together with AMPK, the benefit can only be stronger.

Of all the consumables that I list here, green tea is the most accessible one that will actually make a difference in your autophagy. Green tea helps autophagy because of its active ingredient, EGCG. It is particularly helpful in making autophagy turn on for the liver. Since your liver's health is so important for the general health of your body, drinking green tea every day could make a real difference in living heather and longer.

We also have ginger. Ginger's active ingredient is called 6-shogaol, a chemical that keeps cells in your lungs from being produced too much. This may not be intuitive, but this is actually good for your lungs because it can keep cancer cells from growing too quickly in your lungs, staving off lung cancer. In the meantime, the autophagy you are turning on can clear the chemicals in your lungs that led to cancer cells in the first place.

If you aren't consuming caffeine already, you should really consider it. In specific, caffeine is known to lower your risk for neurodegeneration, which is one of the biggest perks of turning on autophagy. Since you are already getting the process started with autophagy, you might as well maximize your benefits by consuming caffeine.

You won't get autophagy to happen to a satisfactory level with green tea and turmeric alone, but it will help. That goes for all the food items in this chapter. They are not meant to replace all the other big lifestyle changes that will really bring about autophagy. They just help out a lot in making autophagy be the best it can be.

You are not likely to have missed the buzz about CBD oil. If you did, I could fill you in now. CBD is one of the two cannabinoids from the cannabis plant, sometimes referred to as marijuana. However, unlike the other cannabinoid, THC, CBD does not make you high at all. In fact, it does quite the opposite.

Since the cannabis plant was controversial for so long, the research on THC's sister CBD is admittedly limited. However, we do know that CBD leads to less inflammation in the body. CBD even boosts the connections in your brain related to autophagy.

These foods are also great because they are beneficial to your health even outside of autophagy, green tea, and turmeric included.

Our next autophagy-helping food is the reishi mushroom. In the lab, the reishi mushroom was shown to suppress colon cancer cells. This is an interesting case because while there are actually studies showing that autophagy can make cancer cells grow more (cancer cells go through autophagy more), the reishi mushroom has a chemical that stimulates the autophagy of cells that fight against these cancer cells. In most cases, the cancer cells will stop the non-cancer cells from growing, but the reishi mushroom makes sure this doesn't occur.

Coupling fasting with a proper diet in your non-fasting window allows you to cover all your bases with autophagy. Your green tea can increase the potential of autophagy, while turmeric makes it easier to turn on; the reishi mushroom prevents cancer cells from stopping the autophagy of non-cancer cells. These are all things that wouldn't be possible without a proper diet of autophagy-helping foods.

Here are some other foods that you should think about adding to your eating habits: peppers, mushrooms, vinegar, berries, and broccoli. All of these will help you in getting the most possible out of autophagy.

You don't want to only think about autophagy when you pick your foods to eat, though. You still have to think about what is good for your body, after all. Of course, this is not an easy task to do. Plenty of people seem to think they know exactly what you are supposed to eat, despite the fact that everyone knows how much debate there is about what we should eat.

That said, there are some things that we know for sure your body needs, and those are the things we should focus on. A lot of the obvious part is what you should not be eating. Everyone knows not to eat a diet filled with pancakes, Pop-tarts, and chocolate. This is because these foods are filled with calories, which negatively affect your health when consumed in large quantities.

We know of some foods that are always good to choose, like vegetables, unsaturated fats, and a small amount of fruit.

I have told you before that you need to reduce the amount of carbohydrates you have in your diet, but you should also watch the amount of calories you have in general. This will ensure that you will be going in the right direction for your health and body.

Nonetheless, I don't want to lead you to believe that calories are bad, as some do. There is nothing bad about calories in general. In fact, you need calories. It is just that a lot of people forget that it is the nutrients that come from your food that are the most important.

For most people living in the developed world, it is a good idea to try to eat fewer calories, though. Your body has to break down all of the food you eat. Everything that you consume has an effect on your body and your mind. You will fast for less and less time the more calories you eat since you are not able to go through autophagy while your body is digesting. Think about that next time you are about to eat a lot of calories at once.

While you shouldn't only be thinking about foods that turn on autophagy when you decide what to eat, you don't want to eat a lot of foods that slow down autophagy, either. As you know, carbs are your enemy when it comes to getting autophagy going. Your friends are foods that are rich in nutrients.

You also have to make sure your diet has many different kinds of foods. Whether you are fasting to turn on autophagy or not, you can't be healthy without eating all sorts of different foods.

On that note, take the example of craving dessert after eating. Have you ever wondered why there always seems to be room for dessert? The answer to that question is actually three very scientific-sounding words: sensory-specific satiety.

Scientists have been studying people's eating habits in a quest to understand the answer to this conundrum. It turns out that our body has a mechanism to get us a eat many different types of foods. This is meant to prevent us from eating a lot of one food without getting other nutrients from different sources.

Your body tells you to eat ice cream after you say you are full-on one food because of sensory-selective satiety. Hunger can feel like an objective measure of how much you can be eating, but this phenomenon shows us that it is not as black and white as all that. Hunger tells us to eat different kinds of food when we eat too much of one thing. Unfortunately, we have not yet evolved to crave only healthy foods and to avoid unhealthy ones, but this is still a useful mechanism to get us to do what is good for us by not eating only one food.

It is also vital that you make sure to get plenty of Vitamin D from whatever source you can. Vitamin D is essential to a lot of things that our bodies do, and autophagy is one of them. You may not even realize how important Vitamin D is. If you don't get sufficient Vitamin D, there are very real and significant consequences for your autophagy. As a result, the autophagy that you go through will not detox your cells nearly as well as they should.

The good thing is that it is easy to get plenty of this important Vitamin by getting plenty of sun. The sun will provide all of this vitamin that you will need, so if you live somewhere where it is sunny most of the time, this won't be a problem for you. As long as you are sure to use sunscreen to protect your epidermis from harmful ultraviolet rays, you will be safe and get the exposure of Vitamin D that your autophagy requires. If you don't live somewhere sunny, there are still other ways to get Vitamin D.

You can get Vitamin D from a lot of different foods, including milk, or you can even take a supplement for it. However, as you know, we always recommend that you get your vitamins from a food source rather than from a supplement.

One of the reasons that all of the foods we listed are good for your autophagy is that they lower your energy levels. This may not sound like a good thing at first. After all, one of the main perks of turning on autophagy is supposed to be having higher energy levels.

In this context, I am referring to lowering the energy levels of your cells, which is something that all of your cells do. When this happens, your cells have a great chance of entering a state of stress, and you know what that leads to.

As a result, your cells will start breaking down their damaged organelles, proteins, and foreign toxins. Not only that, but every food mentioned in this chapter is particularly healthy for your neurons. Everyone wants to make sure to keep up the health of their brain, so this is a great benefit to have.

We have not yet gotten to the importance of healthy, unsaturated fats in a diet of someone who wants to turn on autophagy. People who start going into ketosis from the keto diet go through a great amount of autophagy when they are sleeping, and it is all because their systems are filled with these healthy fats.

Why exactly are healthy fats such an important part of your new diet? It is because unsaturated fats do the important work of absorbing nutrients like vitamins and minerals. Fats also help in constructing membranes and membranes that protect your nerves from damage. In addition to that, your fats help you move your muscles, keep your blood from clotting, and prevent inflammation in your body.

I have mentioned that unsaturated fats are healthy, and saturated fats are not, but it's time that you learned how exactly that works. Not all fats are created equally. The healthy fats that you want to get plenty of are called polyunsaturated and monounsaturated fats. These fats are always good (unless, of course, you go to extremes, which is always the case with nutrition).

Next, we have trans fats. Trans fats are now banned in many countries, including the United States. The reason they are so harmful is that they provide no health benefit whatsoever while leading to clogging in the blood and an increased risk of inflammation. Trans fat does not occur in nature, either; it is actually the byproduct of artificial processes used to package and preserve food. Clearly, you don't want any trans-fat in your diet.

Finally, our last fat is the saturated fats. If we had to say they were good or bad, we would say that saturated fats are basically bad. However, it is not as if it is poisonous, so it is OK to have a little bit of saturated fat. You just don't want to eat more than a small amount of it, and you probably don't even want to eat it every day.

The worst types of fats are trans fats and saturated fats, while polyunsaturated and monounsaturated fats are the healthy ones that you should eat.

Nutritionists say that around one-third of your calories should come out of good fats like polyunsaturated and monounsaturated fats. You can see what kinds of fats you are eating by looking at the labels on the foods you eat. Since the goods fats are what you are aiming for, make sure you buy plenty of foods like fatty fish, nuts, seeds, and even veggies. These healthy fats are also found in flaxseed.

Since fish is not a common dish in all settings, it can be surprising for some people that the American Heart Association says we should be eating two meals with fatty fish every single week. Healthy fats are so good for us that we should be going out of our way to get them.

Sadly, trans fats and carbohydrates are a normal part of the American diet. Trans fats may not be legal anymore, but we still see plenty of artificial chemicals on the labels of popular snack foods, and these chemicals are probably no better. It should go without saying that you need to avoid packaged snack foods like the plague. They will hinder your autophagy tremendously. We see these chemicals in pastries, fried goods, sugary icing, saltines, brownies, false butter, and more.

What makes healthy fats so important, though? Your blood starts to cause congestion in our veins and arteries, especially as we age. The role of unsaturated fats is helping to unclog them. If you don't get enough healthy fat in your diet, particularly as we get older, you are looking at higher risks for conditions that are caused by clogged arteries.

When it comes to saturated fats, even though they are not completely bad like trans fats, we still don't want to be eating these fats as much as most of us do. You would be surprised by how much-saturated fats get into your diet without you even thinking about it. Doctors tell us that at most, we should be getting 10% of our calories from saturated fats on a daily basis. If you can, you should aim to eat even less saturated fat.

Trans fats and saturated fats both, to different extents, make your cholesterol go up, make your heart disease risk go up, and clog your veins and arteries. As usual, it is worth mentioning that these risks also go up the older you get. That's why it is essential to pay attention to the kinds of fats you are eating every day.

The diet in Mediterranean culture is famous for being high in unsaturated fat, from olive oil in specific. People living in this area are also famous for having a record-breaking low level of heart disease. They are what led nutritionists to learn more about unsaturated fats, eventually, determine that not all fats are bad. Some are actually vital.

Polyunsaturated fats are common in vegetable oil. Vegetable oil is well known for making your cholesterol go down. Omega-3 fats are also considered a polyunsaturated fat. The thing that makes lowering your saturated fat intake easier is that you can often replace the foods with high saturated fat with foods with high unsaturated fat. Any time you have the option to do this, do it. Your heart and arteries will thank you.

If you are going to start consuming more olive oil for the polyunsaturated fats, you do have to be careful, because not every bottle of olive oil is created equal. There is an unfortunate number of olive oil companies that do not use real, natural ingredients for it, meaning you will not get the health benefits from it that you should.

Polyunsaturated fats are a special case for fats because your body is not able to produce these kinds of fats without consuming them. That, and your body actually needs them for various biological processes.

Meanwhile, saturated and trans fats are terrible for your cholesterol. In higher than low amounts, saturated fats lead to blocked arteries, which puts you at risk for health problems.

Despite the common misconception, the amount of fat that you consume does not affect your risk for diseases like cancer. What does affect your risk of cancer is overweight or obese, and this is more likely to happen if you are consuming too many trans and saturated fats, or if you are consuming too much fat overall.

It would be a disservice to talk about diet in the context of autophagy without talking about the health risks associated with being obese or overweight. If you belong to the demographic of overweight women who have already gone through menopause, you should be aware of this risk, especially. People in this demographic can significantly lower their risks for diseases related to weight by following our advice.

The way that you feel subjectively will start to change as a result of fasting and following this new diet. The reason is that hunger has a strong relationship with blood sugar levels. The more glucose you have in your blood, the less you crave food because your system feels like it has enough of it.

Chapter 7: Metabolic Autophagy in Practice

Now armed with tons of knowledge about autophagy and how to take advantage of its effects on your body, you might still be unsure where to begin. It is understandable; after all, it is a lot of information to take in. That's why this chapter is about starting up metabolic autophagy in practice and how to avoid making the same mistakes many autophagy practitioners make when trying to turn on autophagy. To begin, you should consider how many people start living their lives aware of autophagy but give up on harnessing its potential very fast. The key to using autophagy to its highest potential is to start slow and be consistent.

To begin, you should consider how many people start living their lives aware of autophagy but give up on harnessing its potential very fast. The key to using autophagy to its highest potential is to start slow and be consistent.

But we have already discussed the importance of having the right mindset when learning about water fasting. Still, there is one component of turning on autophagy that you cannot underestimate, or you will regret it. And that is sleep.

Sleep is so important to autophagy that it is the first topic in the chapter about turning on autophagy in practice. Even outside the context of autophagy, sleep is a mysterious thing. Not even scientists or psychologists know what it is for. They have guessed that it is for the brain rather than the body, but other than that, they do not know why we even do it.

While sleeping alone doesn't turn on autophagy, you truly shouldn't underestimate the importance of sleep in getting the most out of it. We want to turn on autophagy for our overall health, too, and sleep is an incredibly important part of our overall health.

If you are not getting eight hours of sleep every night, you are not ready to turn on autophagy whenever you can. That's because missing out on sleep is so bad for you that you might as well not do something healthy like fasting to turn on autophagy.

Sleeping is the most important time of the day for autophagy. This is when your body is fixing all the damage you have accumulated, after all, and since autophagy is necessary any time you are repairing, sleep is a crucial time for it. Another reason that sleep is so important for autophagy is that your body isn't using energy for much else at this point. This makes it a good time for processes like autophagy to take place. You aren't using energy to digest, move, talk, or do anything, so your body can take advantage of that and get as much out of the time as possible.

That means if you aren't getting the recommended eight hours of sleep every night, you are egregiously lowering the amount of work that autophagy could be doing on your body.

And this is not even talking about serious sleep deprivation. If you sleep for only six hours instead of eight, sometimes, this is something you should work on improving, too. But some people get even less sleep than that, and this is a problem. The less sleep you get, the less autophagy you are getting in your body. If you have a habit of doing this over time, this creates problems for your health and immune system.

This is not even to mention all of the negative side effects of sleep deprivation that are unrelated to autophagy. Being short on sleep leads to cravings, a lack of clarity of thought, low executive functioning control, and a less efficient metabolism.

To keep things elegant, you should try to think of your time sleeping every night as doing the opposite work of eating during the day. If you spend 4 hours during the day eating, your body spends 8 hours a day breaking all of that down at night.

Depending on the nutritional value of the food, your number of hours breaking down food in autophagy every night could be different, but the point is that your body has to take care of all the chemicals you put in it. This is what your eight hours of sleep are for, and if you aren't getting them, you are hindering the proper functions of your system in a major way.

The complementary period of time to your sleep is what happens when you get up in the morning. While you should be breaking down your food from the previous day in autophagy while you sleep, the next morning, you should eat more than you eat for the rest of the day.

This is not a common thing to do in all cultures, but it is actually the smartest thing to do because your body is better at breaking food down in the morning and earlier in the day.

If you want to go above and beyond, you should really try to go to bed earlier on days that you do a serious fast. If you go to bed early and on an empty stomach, you will be optimizing the autophagy in your cells.

I recommend going to bed earlier because this will help you have more deep sleep or REM sleep. Most of the autophagy that occurs while you are asleep happens during this phase of sleep, so you should try to get as much deep sleep as possible.

Finally, try to maximize the amount of melatonin in your brain when you sleep. Melatonin is essential for turning on autophagy in your brain cells, giving you yet another reason to prioritize sleep if you care about autophagy.

That means it makes the most sense to fit in as many nutrients as you can in the morning, so your stomach can break them down efficiently.

It can be hard to get a good night's sleep these days for a variety of reasons. Back when we lived in caves, we didn't have these problems because the sun went down and we all simply had no choice but to go to bed and wait for the light to come back.

Since we have so many things to do and so many bright lights competing for our attention, getting to bed at a reasonable hour has become an increasingly more difficult task.

Studies show that the blue lights emanating from our screens are detrimental to our sleep. If you care about the quality of your sleep, and if you care about getting to sleep at a reasonable time, you need to find a way to manage the blue lights around you at night. Ideally, you don't interact with your smartphone or laptop at all before you hit the hay.

The next time the sun goes down, I challenge you to accept that to mean it is night time, meaning you don't look at any screens after that happens. You will find that this is almost impossible to do these days. It doesn't help that a lot of us have our work on these gadgets too.

Since it is so hard to deal with blue lights the ideal way, you may have to compromise so you can still sleep as well as you can for your autophagy. If you wear glasses, you can wear special lenses that block out some of the blue light from devices. You can also adjust brightness settings, making your screens darker or sometimes even turning off blue light entirely.

The important thing to know is that if you don't look at these screens before bed, you will see a big difference in the quality of your sleep.

What to Avoid in Your First Fast

Since you are reading a book about fasting before you do it, you get the privilege of learning from other people's mistakes before making these mistakes on your own. Don't make the same mistakes other people make, because you can learn from them now and avoid them later.

Of course, you are bound to make some of the same mistakes. We are all just human. However, equipped with the experiences of others, you can do your best not to repeat the same mistakes.

One big mistake that almost everyone makes does not have long enough fasts. Don't forget that fact we talked about earlier in the book: if you eat a low-carb meal before your fast, you are still digesting it for four hours afterward; if you have a meal with a good amount of carbs before fasting, it takes 8 hours to digest. While you are digesting, you are not in autophagy.

It seems that very few autophagy practitioners are aware of this very helpful fact. They believe they are fasting for 12 hours, but they are really fasting for 8. If they are really out of the loop and not avoiding carbs, that 12-hour fast turns into a 4-hour fast. This little principle can really change the way you think about your fasts.

Of course, there is still value to these shorter fasts, given that you are not eating 4 hours before bed. If you get full autophagy during a full night of sleep, in addition to getting autophagy during the day, you are still doing good by your body. It doesn't matter if it only calculates to be a 4-hour fast after digestion — even that will have a positive effect on your health.

But this is where the value of the water fast really shines because once you become aware of this harsh mathematical reality, you might wish to get more out of your fasting.

All things considered, I would say that short fasts may not be a common mistake, but rather a common opportunity for improvement. You could settle for the daily 4-hour fast with intermittent fasting, but you could also go for more and try to do a 24-hour water fast every other week. You know everything you need to know to do it after reading — what's stopping you from trying?

There are writers on this subject who say that there is no reason to fast for more than 12 hours. However, scientific studies on the matter don't support this idea. In fact, research shows that those who go for 24 hours fasting had 300% more autophagosomes in their bodies. When they went for 12 hours longer, autophagosomes went up 20% more.

As you can see, the number of autophagosomes (and therefore, the level of autophagy) increases astronomically 24 hours into a fast. This level of autophagosomes reaches its highest point at 36 hours, but it doesn't increase nearly as much as it did before.

Again, though, that doesn't mean there is no reason to fast for longer than 24 or 36 hours. Your cells are breaking down toxins and rebuilding cell structures the entire time that you are doing autophagy, so you are still getting this benefit. And as you stay in this level of autophagy for longer, you really notice a difference in how you feel, compared to just going through autophagy when you sleep.

Your takeaway here should be that the biggest increase in autophagy happens after 24 hours of fasting, while the highest level of autophagy happens at 36 hours. You should memorize this fact and take your own health status and goals into consideration to decide the way you want to fast.

As we said before, you will definitely see improvements in your health even if you only do a daily 12-hour fast. I am only telling you about how much more autophagy you get from 24 hours so you can get some perspective, and perhaps to convince you to challenge yourself with a water fast, if your body can safely handle it.

Although your autophagosomes do not increase as nearly as much after 24 hours, you will still continue to be at a very high caliber of autophagy that will do your body a lot of good. Your cells will continue to be detoxified the whole time.

So the first big mistake people make is doing fasts that are too short. The next big mistake is not doing fasts frequently enough. People who make this mistake seem to think that doing a few very intense fasts every year is going to make their bodies healthy, but they are wrong. Once again, I have to repeat that consistency is everything when we are talking about autophagy.

Consistency isn't just about turning on autophagy every day, either. It also means being consistent in your health, and not just expecting one healthy thing that you do to turn on autophagy is going to be enough to make you a healthy individual. Sleep was our example earlier: what is the point of someone who fasts for autophagy if they are running off of six hours of sleep every night? That person still isn't healthy.

You may have an idea of the next aspect of health I am going to bring up in regard to consistency: exercise. It truly seems like exercise is the very last thing that anyone wants to do, but it is extremely good for you to get regular exercise. There is even some solid evidence to suggest that exercise rivals fasting in terms of turning on autophagy the most effectively.

We have an entire chapter devoted to exercising and autophagy, but it is still good to think about it in terms of how it fits together with fasting. No matter if you are overweight, skinny, or athletic, you have to find time to work out on days that you fast. Even if you only work out for fifteen minutes, that's fifteen minutes more of exercise that you didn't have before. That's how valuable exercise is to your health.

Studies on mice have proved the viability of exercise to turn on autophagy. When mice were running in the lab, and scientists measured their level of autophagosomes afterward, they were found to have high levels of autophagosomes after the exercise. Exercises like cardio, therefore, are known to be a good way to turn on autophagy.

Without digging too much into the exercise chapter, there is actually evidence that strength/resistance training is more effective in turning on autophagy than cardio. You can work on your muscles to reduce tissue loss while also turning on autophagy.

It is strange that cardio is always so emphasized since there is a lot of evidence that strength/resistance training could be even better for you. Of course, cardio is great for your body too, but maybe the real reason that cardio gets such a focus is that it is seen as the best way to lose weight.

So far, I have told you to avoid fasting not long enough, avoid not fasting consistently, and to avoid not exercising. You could sum that up as fast for long enough, fast often enough, and don't forget to exercise.

There is another common mistake with fasting that connects to our discussion about the mental aspect of water fasting, as well as to the issue of fasting with consistency. To put it in few words, in order to succeed with intermittent fasting — or any fast, really — you have to resist the temptation to give up.

We said it before: it is easy to start things, but following through with them is another story.

I won't repeat the part about needing to keep a clear goal, but that still applies here. To avoid giving up before you can even start, you need to start out with small goals. You could even call them easy goals. The easiest starting point for intermittent fasting and keeping yourself from eating after dinner at 6pm.

If you do that, a 12-hour fast only requires you to wait until 6am the next morning to eat. (As you know, this is really an 8-hour fast, but for the sake of ease, we will keep calling them their normal lengths without considering digestion.)

Once you have a hang of the shorter fast, you can go for the longer ones.

The key to success and safety with the water fast is going into it with your goals clearly defined. Ask yourself right now, since you are pretty far into the book at this point: what are you doing this for? Do you want to lose weight? Do you want to look younger? Do you want to live longer?

While it's true that autophagy achieves all three for you, you still need to have a purpose for autophagy that is for you and you alone. If you don't, you won't be very likely to change entire aspects of your lifestyle for it. Once you have a well-defined purpose for something, all the rest starts to fall into place, because you know what you want to do.

The opposite of that is when you don't have a well-defined purpose at all, and you give up easily. If you don't know why you're doing something, it is very easy for you to give up on it. You don't even have a point in continuing with it, so why wouldn't you?

It is very easy to start things. Anyone can start a 300-word novel. Anyone can start a sculpture. What makes you accomplished is when you can start something and finish it. Autophagy and water fasting is no different. If you have a clear reason you want to see through your first water fast to the end, you will be far less likely to fall out of it.

Having your goal in mind isn't just a preventive measure against giving up; it's almost a way for you to do things the right way. If you are in the middle of a water fast, you might be tempted to get a snack, even though you know it ruins the purpose of the entire fast. When you already know your goal for water fasting, though, you are a lot less likely to fall for temptations like these.

You can tell yourself, "I am fasting to lose weight. I won't lose weight if I add more food into my stomach during this fast, so I'm not going to cheat on the fast with that cookie."

Alternatively, if you went into your water fast without a goal like this, things would probably go a lot different. You would see the cookie and say, "Well, it is my first day fasting. I can do things the correct way next time." Since you don't have a clear reason for water fasting, there just isn't that emotional weight to cheating on the fast that there otherwise would be.

A second crucial but often overlooked part of the mindset of someone who succeeds in the water fast is knowledge of fasts and autophagy. Plenty of people believe they know things about these topics, so much that they actually do fasting the way they believe is correct, whether it is right or not.

Fortunately, you have this whole book of easy-to-understand information about fasting and autophagy. You could return to it if you need to know more, but chances are, you are absorbing it so well that it isn't even necessary. You already have this second crucial part of the mindset covered.

Finally, there is the third and last part of the mindset required to succeed in a water fast, and it is adaptability. You have lots of goals that propelled you to do a water fast in the first place, but the one that will carry the fate of all the others is your adaptability to a new, healthier way of living. This mental aspect will determine if you continue water fasting a few times a month, or if it is just something you do one time and never again.

You will get some health benefits from the autophagy that comes from water fasting one time, but these benefits are pointless if you don't keep it up. That's why it's so crucial that you adapt well to the new habits you formed and do it again in a few weeks.

Chapter 8: Autophagy and Training to Build Muscle

There is some research to back the claim that resistance training — that is, muscle-building exercises — turn on autophagy in your body even more than fasting. When you are at the gym using your muscles, you are making tiny tears in your muscle tissue that your cells have to repair using the process of autophagy.

A lot of people are hesitant to go to the gym at all, let alone do more intense exercise like resistance training. But if you want to get as much out of your body's autophagy as possible, your efforts are best spent in working out your muscles.

After seven chapters about the food you put into your body, we can finally focus on something that is equally important to autophagy: exercise. We have brought it up again and again, but we have not yet gone in-depth on what makes it such a vital part of turning on autophagy.

Exercise is such an effective method of turning on autophagy that it is perfectly valid to choose it as your main method of doing so. However, most people will not choose to do this because exercising regularly is much harder to keep up than intermittent fasting.

As always, the best option is doing a combination of both: fasting and exercising. If you do your daily 8 hour fast before your run on the treadmill, you will increase your autophagy much more than if you did just one or the other.

If you still aren't sure if exercise isn't important for autophagy, consider the study showing that those who did strength exercises for twenty minutes had higher levels of autophagosomes than those who fasted for 36 hours.

It can be hard to believe, but this is what bearer out in science. This is so hard to accept, since it may be true that mostly no one wants to exercise. How could it be true that exercise is more effective in turning on autophagy than fasting?

It may be a comfort to know that, in a way, fasting is still more effective than normally turning on autophagy through exercising. That's because exercise is a challenging thing to keep doing on a routine basis.

A lot of people get excited about fasting, only to quit eventually. You can imagine how much worse this phenomenon is with working out. If exercise was the way that most people turned on autophagy, hardly anyone would be getting the benefits of it.

Thankfully, we have intermittent fasting available to us as our main path to autophagy. However, since this is a book about doing what is best for our health and our bodies, we still need to at least learn about what exercise can do for our natural detox agent.

Remember that autophagy is not really ever "on" or "off." There is always some autophagy going on in your body, in some organ or another. Talking about "turning on autophagy" is just a simpler way of saying that we want to make your autophagy reach more significant goals for our bodies than it would if we didn't intentionally "turn it on."

This means we are not literally trying to turn on autophagy — it is always on to some degree. It is that degree that we are trying to influence: we want to turn on autophagy to the highest degree possible using fasting, the keto diet, and exercise.

The "regular" level of autophagy is often called the maintenance mode by experts. The maintenance mode is the amount of autophagy that everyone gets, even if they have no clue what autophagy even means.

When we say, "turn on autophagy," we really mean "turn on advanced autophagy." We mean go from maintenance mode autophagy to advanced autophagy.

Fasting alone will certainly get you to the level of advanced autophagy, but you can go even further than that. You will want to once you become enamored by the energy autophagy gives you the weight it helps you lose and the quality of skin that it restores for you.

You shouldn't think that either fasting or exercise is pointless just because one alone will do the trick. Truthfully, you are probably best off picking one or the other in the beginning, so you don't get burnt out. Of course, intermittent fasting is always your best choice to avoid this consequence. But you will have this chapter as a resource to go back to once you start to see the positive effects autophagy has on your body and you want to have even more of it.

The Health of the Individual who Exercises to Increase Autophagy

The average person who exercises regularly probably does not know about autophagy, just like the average person, in general, doesn't know about autophagy. But it's not only the benefits of exercise overall that makes it good for you. Autophagy specifically will see positive consequences as a result of your regular exercise.

For one, in people who exercise, autophagosomes are at much higher counts than people who do not exercise. Scientists saw this in an experiment that paid attention to the autophagy levels of athletes and non-athletes. To no one's surprise, the athletes had more autophagosomes than the control group.

You should be able to look at this from the other side, though. There are benefits to the autophagy that fasting offers that exercise does not. For one, in mice that fasted to turn on autophagy, skeletal muscle fibers were strengthened. The mice could stop their muscle fibers from degrading because autophagy from fasting could stop dysfunctional organelles from building up. Mice who turned on autophagy through exercise did not see this benefit at all.

The point is that fasting and exercise both turn on autophagy, but they don't always turn on the same kind of autophagy. You can't go wrong by turning on autophagy through both means.

Another example has to do with the equilibrium of your muscles when you exercise. It can be hard for your body to keep them at equilibrium, but if you fast, the autophagy that is triggered can greatly help in maintaining equilibrium.

If you fast as well as exercise, you will also see a greater count of collagen in your skin cells, the protein they produce that keeps your skin elastic. If you do only one or the other, you do not see as great of an effect.

It goes to show you that while exercise may be shown to turn on higher levels of autophagy in a shorter amount of time, the autophagy that you are looking for is not always achieved through either means. You don't have to decide on just one; when the time comes that you realize the benefits autophagy gives you, decide to do both.

Maybe the best benefit that combining the two can give you is in dealing with loose skin that can come from weight loss. In a study where people who lost weight with either fasting, exercising, or both, the respondents who said they did both had less loose skin than those who turned on autophagy with just one method or the other.

This loose skin is often referred to as a "skin curtain," and many people will even say that they are hesitant to lose weight because of the threat of loose skin.

There is a lot of misinformation out there about loose skin, so it is understandable that people would be concerned about it. But loose skin doesn't have to be a sure thing; it all depends on how quickly you lose weight, your level of hydration, your level of autophagy, and your age.

Three out of four of these things are completely in your control. If you make sure to drink plenty of water, pace yourself in your exercise routine and fasting, and use all the methods we describe in this book to maximize your autophagy, your loose skin fears won't be as horrible as you might imagine.

The "skin curtain" is often seen in people who lose weight without considering autophagy as part of the equation. You see, autophagy helps against the threat of loose skin because autophagy is all about your cells eating dead cells to use them for raw materials and replace them with new cells. If you are keeping up a healthy level of autophagy while you are losing weight, by the time you lose the weight and your skin has to readjust, it will be able to do so much more easily. All because your cells were taken care of through autophagy. Autophagy keeps your skin tight and youthful, no matter how much weight you lose.

It is surprising that we have not even talked much about skin, yet to this point, but the chapter on exercise is an excellent opportunity to do it. Your skin will truly give off a new glow if you make autophagy a new part of your routine, but this is doubly true if you make exercise a part of your autophagy routine.

At the end of the day, though, skin is usually a matter of cosmetics, much like weight can be. If you are more concerned about your health and risk for age-related disease, exercise is still a good choice for autophagy stimulation. This is because exercise is the best way you can lower the inflammation in your body, pretty close to diet and fasting.

Your inflammation may be pretty high, depending on the healthiness of your previous lifestyle. People who ate poorly before, smoked, were mostly sedentary, or drank a lot are at higher risk of high inflammation. Fortunately, exercise is so powerful that it can reverse inflammation that results from all of these factors. Inflammation is the source of a lot of risks for age-related disease, so reducing it is always a good idea.

Your body overall performs better when you don't have as much inflammation. Chronic inflammation, in particular, is what will make you start to see the beginning symptoms of different age-related diseases.

Exercise doesn't have to be as painful as you might envision it to be in your mind. Just like with fasting, you have to start small and work your way up to more ambitious goals.

Keep your goals written down in a notebook that you can look at every day. Do this from the very beginning, so you don't lose sight of what you are trying to do with autophagy and exercise.

Your first task is to follow through with the first action step of your fitness plan. If you can follow through with it for a few weeks, this is when you start to work towards higher goals.

We said that you might go from an 8-hour fast to a 10-hour fast. With exercise, the situation is almost the same. You might start out telling yourself to go to the gym once a week for thirty minutes (or less, depending on your level of fitness). After you are able to follow through with this small goal for a few weeks, write down that you want to go to the gym for thirty minutes twice a week. Once you can follow through with the second goal consistently for a few weeks, build on that one. You get the idea; you have to start small with your goals if you expect to actually achieve them.

Finally, you have to think about what kind of exercise you are going to do. There are experts who tell you there are a dozen different kinds of ways to work out, but to keep things simple, we can really say there are just three: cardio, core, and resistance.

Cardio is running, biking, endurance, and so on. These are exercises that test the capacity of your lungs and how long you can strain yourself physically. There have been tests on mice that show they went through significant autophagy because of cardio, so this is a valid way to go.

Core exercises are less tested in the context of autophagy, but we know that physical activity, in general, is good for autophagy, so we can basically assume it turns on autophagy as well.

Finally, we have resistance training. Some people call this strength training. Resistance training is all about using your muscles, lifting weights, and increasing your strength. There is actually valid new research suggesting that resistance training is the best method of turning on autophagy out of all of them.

Cardio was demonstrated to make the number of autophagosomes in mice go up, but resistance training was demonstrated to make autophagy turn on even more. This means that working on your muscles is probably the best way to turn on autophagy.

Of course, we still have to consider practicality. Practicality is what makes intermittent fasting still take the cake when it comes to the best way to turn on autophagy, just because far more people are going to be willing to abstain from eating for hours a day than are work on their arms every other day.

Resistance training is so good for autophagy because it puts your cells through long periods of stress, especially in your muscles cells. When your cells are in this state, they go into their resources of cellular garbage to get energy. If you do resistance training exercises over time, your cells are going through high levels of autophagy for a long period of time, and it really gets your autophagosomes to come out.

Not only that, but this kind of autophagy will keep you from seeing as much muscle loss as you get older. When you have more muscle mass, this is an indication that you have better general health; when you are in better shape already, your autophagy is better too. This is why resistance training is so effective in turning on this natural detoxifier.

You may be familiar with the relaxed feeling you get after you do strength exercises. Part of this feeling is the rush of endorphins you get in your brain, as these are your body's natural pain relievers. But the other reason for this feeling is from the tiny tears that you make in your muscles when you use them.

The kind of stress that resistance training puts you in is the perfect kind for turning on autophagy: short-term acute stress. The most straightforward way to achieve it is by simply lifting weights. If you think you can take it, you would be doing yourself a great service by doing weight lifting every day for about 30 minutes. That may seem like a lot, but the benefits your body would reap from it would far outweigh the negatives you feel from doing it.

A Note before the Conclusion

There are many things that make the autophagy-centered lifestyle different from other health practices. One of them is the simplicity of doing it. When you follow the keto diet, the only things you need to pay attention to on the nutritional label are carbohydrates and the kinds of fats. Compared to other diets, this requires very little of you.

Fasting is even simpler. You don't have to count calories, because you have to stay away from them completely. I'm not saying this is easy, but the hard rule of "don't eat for 24 hours" is very straightforward.

Fasting can be hard for people at first, but you will probably be surprised. People tend to find it to be easier than they expected.

If you fail at your first fast, consider shortening your goal, from 16 hours to 12 hours, for example. There is no rush in developing your fasting routine. When you induce autophagy, you are going the extra mile for your body. Be proud of yourself for that and let yourself take it slow.

Sometimes the mind can seem like a mystical thing that is impossible to understand, so let's touch briefly on your brain and how it fits into building these new habits.

Much like autophagy, the study of the brain has made great progress in the past decade. Now we know that the cells in your brain (called neurons) are connected to one another with trillions of connections, called synapses.

This is a tremendous discovery. The discovery of synapses tells us that the connections in our brain change constantly, depending on the inputs we give it. If you create new habits like fasting once a week, eating new foods, and exercising regularly, you are creating new connections in your brain. Once these connections have been solidly established (which takes about a month or so, just like a habit), living your life a new way will just feel normal.

Conclusion

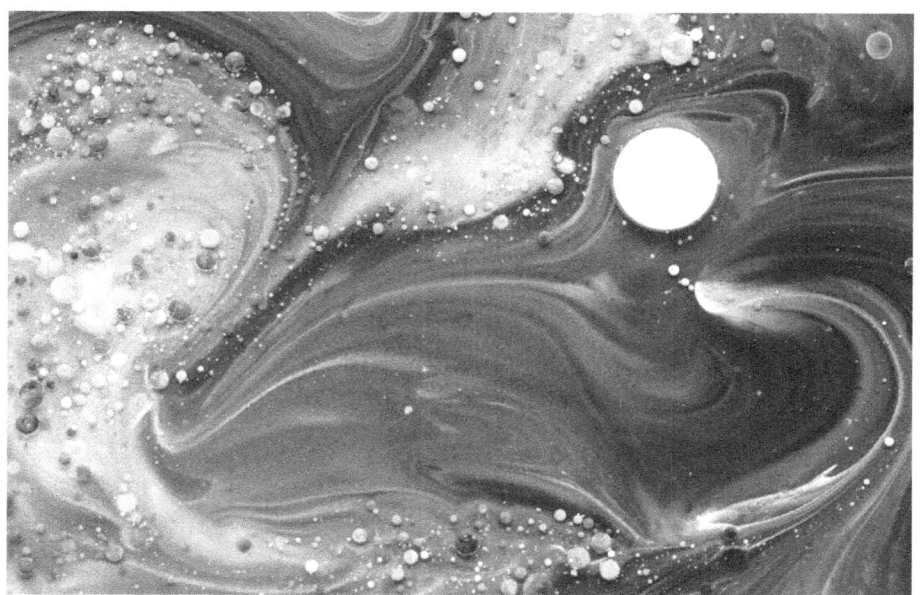

Thank you for making it through to the end of *Autophagy*, let's hope it was informative and able to provide you with all of the tools you need to achieve your goals whatever they may be.

Scientists are not finished making discoveries about the potential healing powers of autophagy, but they have found out enough about this biological process to tell us that turning on autophagy in your body is a great thing to do for your health. The health of your cells is the health of your body, so keeping your cells free of toxins and thus running more smoothly has all sorts of positive health consequences. People who turn on autophagy have lower inflammation, weigh less, have lower blood pressure, and have generally better biomarkers.

For most people, intermittent fasting is the best option for turning on your autophagy. You have read about the variety of techniques that will also have this effect on your body, but intermittent fasting is the most practical one for several reasons. If you made exercise your main path to achieving autophagy, it is more likely than not, you would fall out of your workout routine and lose all the benefits of autophagy. If the keto diet was your main path towards regular autophagy, there is a good chance that you would not keep this up either.

You won't run into this issue with intermittent fasting because it requires nothing but a small adjustment in your day-to-day life: the time that you eat. With all that said, you should absolutely shoot for exercising and dieting in a way to turn on autophagy in addition to intermittent fasting. I am only recommending intermittent fasting as a jumping-off point. Once you are in the routine of fasting, you will probably feel motivated to maximize your body's natural detoxifier in other ways, too.

I hope this book has helped you learn how to aim for higher things for your health and body. If you are curious to learn more about the science of autophagy, look no further than the appendix at the back of the book.

Finally, if you found this book useful in any way, a review on Amazon is always appreciated!

From the same Author

Intermittent Fasting Diet Guide: *A Complete Step-By-Step Guide for Heal Your Body, Weight Loss, Fat Burn and Live in a Healthy and Happy Way with the Autophagy Process*

(Meal Plan with 60 Recipes).

Cook, J. (2019 Nov 17).

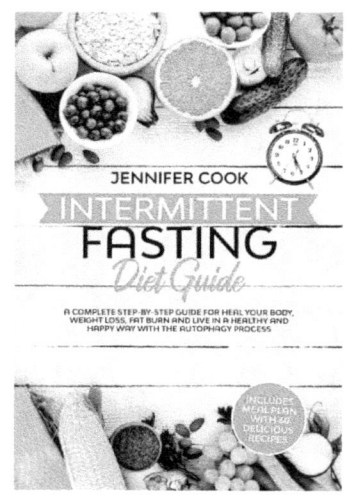

Intermittent Fasting for Women 101: *The Ultimate Step-by-Step Guide for Weight Loss, Even If You Are Over 50, with the Keto Diet, 16/8 Method and Self-Cleansing Through the Metabolic Process of Autophagy.*

Cook, J. (2019 Dec 31).

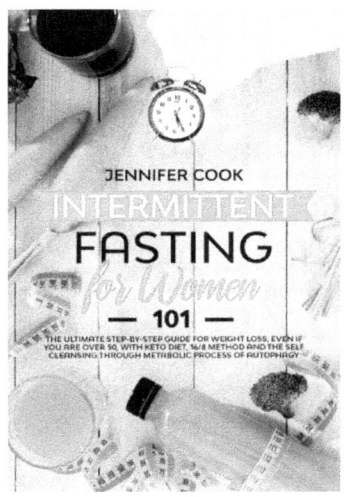

Appendix:
Scientific studies on autophagy, intermittent fasting and related subjects

Alirezaei, Kemball, Flynn, Wood, Whitton Kiosses. *Short-term fasting induces profound neuronal autophagy*. Published online 2010 Aug 14.

ncbi.nlm.nih.gov/pmc/articles/PMC3106288/

The researchers in this study watched the autophagosomes — collectors of material to be broken down in autophagy — of cells of people who fasted. They found that the number of autophagosomes increased significantly in people who fasted and that as a result, they had an increase of autophagy in their brains. Autophagy is known to have a profoundly beneficial effect on the brain in the context of neurodegenerative disease.

Finnell, Saul, Goldhamer, Myers. *Is fasting safe? A chart review of adverse effects during medically supervised, water-only fasting.* Published 2018 February 20. ncbi.nlm.nih.gov/pmc/articles/PMC5819235/

The article starts out conceding that water fasting has been proved to have some health benefits. The author felt there was a lack of research on potential negative consequences of water fasting, which is the subject of this experiment. The conclusion after testing patients on water fasting was that it was safe enough to use as treatment in a controlled setting.

Francoise, Grundler, Bergouignan, Dorinda, Michalsen. *Safety, health improvement, and well-being during a 4 to 21-day fasting period in an observational study including 1422 subjects.* Published 2019 Jan 2. ncbi.nlm.nih.gov/pmc/articles/PMC6314618/

This study aims to study subjects who are not obese who do fasting over a long period of time. The main measurements were the health changes of the subject as well as their safety over the span of a year. Even over the course of a year, there were significant and measurable differences in weight, waist size, and blood pressure. The subjects increased improved well-being, both physically and emotionally. They expressed a diminished feeling of hunger as well. Fewer than 1% expressed safety concerns from the experiment, and over 80% said they noticed improvements in health.

Ganesan, Habboush, Sultan. *Intermittent Fasting: The Choice for a Healthy Lifestyle*. Published online 2018 July 9. ncbi.nlm.nih.gov/pmc/articles/PMC6128599/

Says that the basic reduction of food consumption leads to weight loss. Looked at over 800 studies about intermittent fasting done in the last two decades, and takes note of the fact that only 4 of all of these meet the criteria required to be considered entirely scientific, such as having a control group. Still, the study says that an increase in fat loss was a consistent trend in these studies. IF is determined to be an effective way of losing weight, but says that more research is needed to say any more.

Stockman, Thomas, Burke, Apovian. *Intermittent Fasting: Is the Wait Worth the Weigh?* Published online 2019 June 1.

ncbi.nlm.nih.gov/pmc/articles/PMC5959807/

A meta-study of research done about the effects of intermittent fasting on both animals and humans. Note that IF is difficult to study since many variations of it exist. Says that the results can also vary as a result, although there is a consistent conclusion that IF leads to weight loss and improved biomarker. Even showed that in animals, IF led to less of oxidative stress, better cognition, and slowed aging. Said there were anti-inflammatory effects as well.

Templeman, Gonzalez, Thompson, Betts. *The role of intermittent fasting and meal timing in weight management and metabolic health*. Published 2019 April 26. ncbi.nlm.nih.gov/pubmed/31023390

Centered around the problem of obesity as a public health issue, this study seeks to find solutions, postulating that intermittent fasting may be one. Looks into the effectiveness of fasting in general without assuming that it must be good. They concluded that fasting longer than 16 hours, in particular, showed some physiological difference in the people who participated, including fat loss and insulin control. The paper says that the reason for this change could be caloric restriction rather than fasting.

www.ingramcontent.com/pod-product-compliance
Lightning Source LLC
Chambersburg PA
CBHW070639220526
45466CB00001B/227